"Nature has provided our bodies with everything we need to survive.
With a balanced diet and positive mindset, we can learn to thrive.."
Monty's Dream's

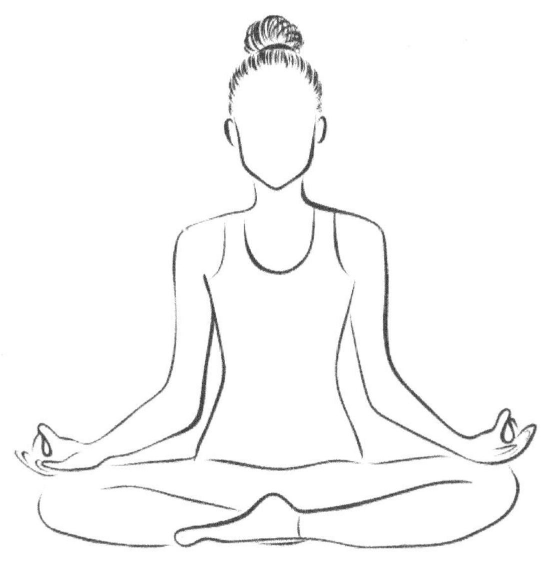

https://healthhearty.com/gout-diet-foods-to-eat

https://www.healthline.com/nutrition/best-diet-for-gout#TOC_TITLE_HDR_3

https://elevatehealthaz.com/wp-content/Purine%20Table.pdf

https://med.virginia.edu/ginutrition/wp-content/uploads/sites/199/2014/04/Low-Fructose.pdf

https://www.mayoclinic.org/diseases-conditions/gout/symptoms-causes/syc-20372897

https://www.arthritis.org/health-wellness/healthy-living/nutrition/healthy-eating/gout-diet-dos-and-donts

https://www.cdc.gov/arthritis/basics/gout.html

https://www.niams.nih.gov/health-topics/gout#tab-overview

https://www.medicalnewstoday.com/articles/144827#types

https://www.arthritis.org/diseases/gout

https://www.onmanorama.com/lifestyle/health/2019/01/24/super-coriander-the-leaf-that-can-lower-uric-acid-creatinine-levels.html

https://www.healthline.com/nutrition/top-10-evidence-based-health-benefits-of-turmeric#TOC_TITLE_HDR_3

Disclaimer

The information contained in this book is provided for general purposes only. It is not intended as and should not be relied upon as medical advice. Do not diagnose or medicate yourself without first seeking medical advice.

The publisher and author are not responsible for any specific health needs that may require medical supervision. If you have any health problems or have any doubts about anything contained in this book, you should contact a qualified medical, dietary or other appropriate professional. The publisher and author do not accept responsibility for any loss, harm or damage that may result as a misuse of this book or your failure to seek appropriate medical advice.

The publisher and author make no representations or warranties with respect to the accuracy or completeness of the contents of this work. The content in this book may not be suitable for everyone. This work is sold with the understanding that the publisher and author is not engaged in rendering medical, legal or other professional advice. Images and photos in this work is used as inspiration only.

That fact an individual, organization or website is referred to in this work is a citation and/or a potential source of further information does not mean that the publisher or author endorses the individual, organization or website. Furthur readers should be aware that websites listed in this work may have changed or disappeared since this work was written and when this book was read.

Welcome!

I'm Jade Patterson

In this book, you will find recipes that I make for the people I love. Healthy, gout-friendly, and tasty.

As a sufferer of gout myself, I find these work for me.

However, I recommend you do what works best for you and your family.

Table of Contents

I. INTRODUCTION

BREAKFAST AND BRUNCH

Table of Contents

BREAKFAST AND BRUNCH

LUNCH AND LIGHT MEALS

Table of Contents

Table of Contents

Table of Contents

Introduction

The body is designed to carry out all its functions optimally and stave off external attacks from toxins and pathogens without outside help apart from the food you eat.

A healthy body relies on natural and unprocessed food. This was easily achievable in the days of our ancestors.

Food has undergone a rapid metamorphosis in the last 10,000 years, from wild-grown food to naturally farmed food, then the agricultural revolution to genetically modified food and processed foods.

Our digestive system has not been able to catch up, explaining some of the exponential increase of chronic illnesses. Our bodies may look at some processed foods as an external attack and launch a retaliatory response that repeatedly happens because we keep eating the same foods, which leads to chronic inflammation and a host of autoimmune conditions.

Today we face the challenge of instant food, processed foods, and a sedentary lifestyle that have contributed significantly to making us sicker. Considering this, it is vital to take care of your mind, body, and soul as this provides you with many long-term benefits such as:

- Being filled with vitality
- Improving your mental, physical and emotional health
- Allowing you to stay in control of your life
- You may live longer
- Lowering the risk of heart disease, type 2 diabetes, and some cancers
- You get to enjoy and appreciate your life
- You become a role model for your children, family, and friends

Staying healthy in the 21st century takes work, unlike the days of our ancestors where everything they ate was natural. Today you must always consider what you eat because unhealthy processed foods surround us.

Our environment and technological advances encourage a sedentary lifestyle. Today's kids no longer play outside; instead, they prefer to play video games all day.

This book focuses on providing information about gout and offers practical guidelines on how to manage it as well as how to lead a healthy lifestyle that is applicable for the rest of your life. These guidelines are not just limited to gout patients and can be shared with your family, friends or anyone interested in adopting a healthy lifestyle.

We will be shedding light on what you need to do and watch out for to lead a high-quality life despite having a gout diagnosis.

So please put on your reading glasses and join me on this incredible health journey!

Behind The Curtain

If you are reading this book, you will undoubtedly have tried many different remedies promising a cure for gout. You may even have succumbed to trying some of the old wives' tales endorsing all sorts of weird and wonderful ways to achieve gout relief.

It's fair to assume that none of these options proved helpful or viable, at least long term, and that is why you are now reading this book.

The good news is, you have made the right decision and what is about to be revealed is the gateway to a new you. It is a must for anyone who wants to be healthy, regardless of whether they suffer from gout-related health issues. The content applies to everyone and anyone who aspires to be healthy. It's that simple.

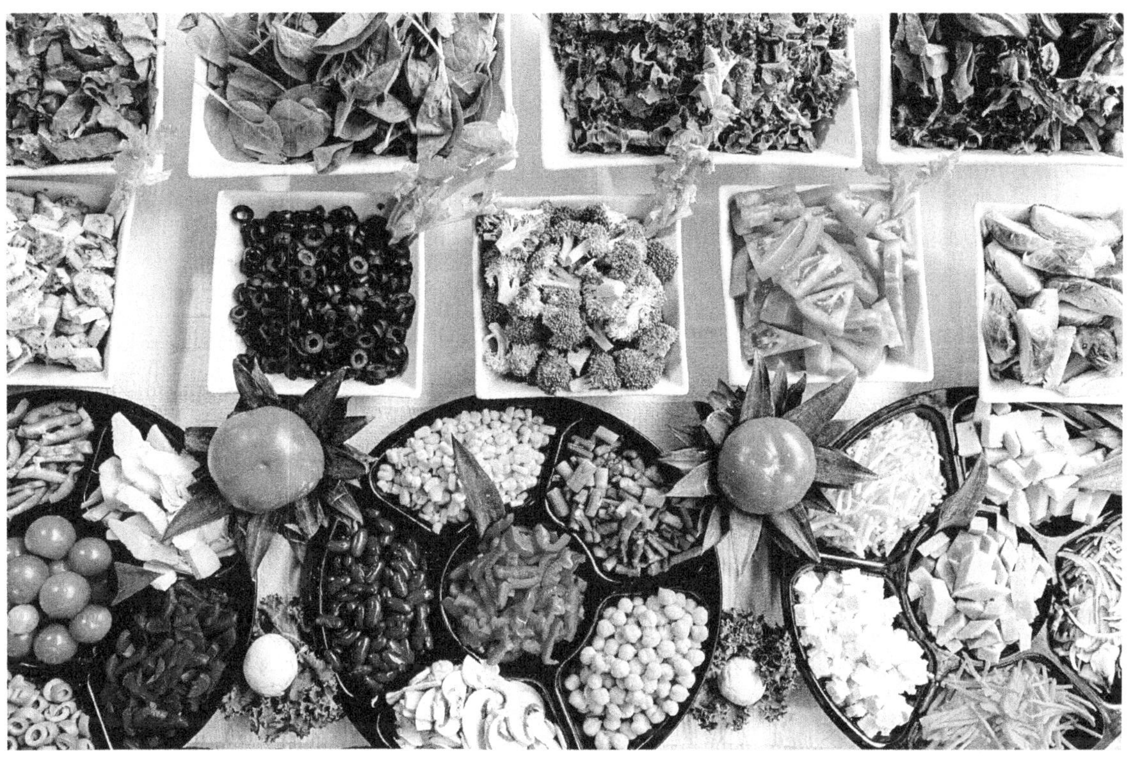

What is Gout?

Gout is a form of arthritis that can be extremely painful. Gout affects 2-3 adults in every 100 people, making it one of the most common forms of arthritis.

Historically, it was believed that gout was self-inflicted, too much rich living like the kings of our past, such as King Henry VIII.

However, recent studies have revealed this is not the case. While diet may play a part in making gout attacks more likely, for the most part, gout is most likely genetic or related to other health issues.

Both men and women are affected by gout, though women are more likely to experience gout after menopause.

Gout typically happens suddenly, causing extreme pain in the joints.

For most people, gout occurs in the big toe, but it can also affect the feet, ankles, fingers, wrists, or knees. The joint typically appears red, swollen, and tender.

It is unclear why gout is most common in the foot or big toe joint. Some studies believe it could be related to injuries and osteoarthritis.

Once a gout attack occurs, it is usually at its most painful within 12-24 hours. Episodes can last a few days to a few weeks, and often they will start to get better even without treatment. It is believed that this happens because the cells of the immune system stop reacting to the uric acid crystals; in turn, the inflammation reduces. However, most people will need short-term pain and inflammation treatment to help reduce the severity of the attack.

Gout flare-ups occur intermittently until such a point when the inflammation becomes persistent and turns chronic. After years of acute gout inflammation, the MSU (monosodium urate) crystals may collect in tendons and joints. Some people may notice the build-up of these crystals under the skin, often referred to as tophi. These usually appear under the skin around the knuckles, fingers, ears, elbows, and feet.

What causes gout?

Contrary to the belief that gout is a rich man's disease, gout is caused by higher-than-normal uric acid in the bloodstream.

Uric acid occurs when our body breaks down purines.

Some uric acid arises from the breakdown of purines from food. But most will come from the natural breakdown of purines in the cells of our body.

As the uric acid builds up, the kidneys will usually remove the surplus, passing it out the body as urine.

If the body is producing too much uric acid or the kidneys don't remove enough, it can build up, turning into tiny crystals in the joints. These crystals in the joints are what cause the pain, swelling, and tenderness that people with gout experience. High levels of uric acid may also increase the risk of cardiovascular disease.

Genetic predisposition
Lots of scientific research has shown that gout is hereditary. In fact, one in five patients with gout has a close relative who also suffers from gout.

Diet

Uric acid is a by-product of the process of breaking down purines. Eating foods that are high in purines that can result in uric acid build-up in your body can lead to gout.

However, research has shown that there is one exception to the rule. High-purine vegetables do not trigger gout attacks.

But interestingly, high fructose and sugar-sweetened drinks can increase the risk of gout attacks, even though they maybe be low in purines.

Low-fat dairy products, soy products, and high vitamin C have been shown to help prevent gout attacks by reducing blood uric acid levels.

Health conditions

Diagnosed or undiagnosed underlying health conditions can significantly increase your risk of developing gout. These include:

- Diabetes
- Obesity
- High blood pressure
- Kidney disease
- Osteoarthritis
- Psoriasis

Medication

Some medications increase the amount of uric acid in your body, which increases your risk of developing gout.

These include:

- Niacin, which is often used to treat high cholesterol levels
- Diuretics used to reduce fluid build-up in your body and to treat high blood pressure
- Ciclosporin, used to treat psoriasis
- Beta-blockers and ACE inhibitors often used to treat high blood pressure
- Some drugs administered during chemotherapy
- Low dose aspirin that's used to reduce the risk of blood clots

Diagnosis of Gout

Before a doctor can conclude that a patient has gout, they will try to eliminate all other possible reasons for swelling, including inflammation, kidney failure, congestive heart failure, infections, or a blood clot. Your physician will go over your medical history then talk to you about your symptoms. However, it is important to note that it is difficult to give a gout diagnosis based solely on the symptoms you are presenting, as other forms of arthritis can present with the same symptoms.

To help get a precise diagnosis of gout, your physician may:

- Do a joint fluid test that involves using a syringe needle to extract some of the fluid from your affected joint, to check for any uric acid crystals.

- Run a blood test to check the amount of uric acid in your blood. However, it is important to note that a blood test can be misleading as some people have high uric acid levels but don't develop gout, while others have all of the symptoms of gout apart from high uric acid levels.
- Do an ultrasound, x-ray or a CT scan on your joints to get a clear picture of what is going on.

Treatment of Gout

It's advisable to seek treatment within twenty-four hours of experiencing a gout flare-up, as your doctor will be able to provide you with the best treatment option before the condition progresses. There are two main types of medication that are used to address two different problems.

The first type of medication is designed to address the pain and inflammation associated with a gout flare-up, while the second type of medication is designed to lower the levels of uric acid, thus preventing gout-related complications.

Your physician will help you determine which form of medication is best suited to the symptoms that you are presenting.

Drugs used to Treat Gout

The medication used to treat gout attacks and also prevent future flare-ups include:

Colchicine

Also known as Colcrys, Mitigare, or Gloperba, this drug is an anti-inflammatory. It is very effective in reducing the pain linked to a gout flare-up. However, many patients complain of side effects such as nausea, diarrhea, and vomiting.

NSAIDs (Nonsteroidal An-inflammatory Drugs)

These include over-the-counter medications such as: Motrin IB and Advil, which are forms of ibuprofen, Aleve, which is naproxen sodium, as well as stronger NSAIDs such as indomethacin (Tivorbex, Indocin) or Celebrex, which is celecoxib. The side effects of NSAIDs include ulcers, bleeding, and stomach pain.

Corticosteroids

These types of medication, such as prednisone, help in relieving pain and inflammation. You can get these in pill form or have them injected into the joint that is suffering from gout. Common side effects of taking corticosteroids include elevated blood sugar levels, blood pressure, and mood changes.

Drugs That Prevent Gout Complications

Depending on the frequency of your gout attacks and the severity of the symptoms during such episodes, your doctor may advise on a certain medication that will help reduce your risk of experiencing gout-related symptoms as well complications.

If you have significant damage caused by gout such as tophi, kidney stones, chronic kidney disease, joint damage visible through x-ray images, your physician will recommend drugs that work to lower the uric acid levels in your body.

These drugs include:

Drugs that boost the elimination of uric acid

Probenecid is prescribed to improve the kidney's efficiency in the elimination of uric acid from the body. The common side effects of this drug are kidney stones, stomach pain, and rashes.

Drugs that inhibit the uric acid synthesis

Allopurinol (Lopurin, Aloprim and Zyloprim) and febuxostat are used to reduce the amount of uric acid produced by your body. These drugs, however, have side effects such as hepatitis, fever, nausea, impaired liver function, heart-related death, rashes, and kidney problems.

How to Prepare for A Doctor's Appointment

It is important that you schedule a doctor's appointment when you start experiencing gout-related symptoms. The earlier you catch it, the better. After your first examination, your physician will more likely refer you to a rheumatologist - a specialist in diagnosing and treating inflammatory joint conditions, including arthritis.

Before this appointment, you should prepare a set of questions as well as any information that is relevant to how you are feeling at the moment.

Some of the things you should do include:

Create a list of your medical history

This will include all health conditions you have ever experienced, even those that you feel are not correlated to the gout-like symptoms you are experiencing. Include all forms of treatment you have previously received, including the drugs prescribed to you and the side effects, if any, that you experienced.

If you have a family history of any of the mentioned conditions, write them down.

Note down all symptoms you are currently experiencing.

This should include: when you first noticed these symptoms, the times they tend to be most severe, and the frequency they occur.

Write down important personal experiences.

It's essential to let the doctor know about any significant experiences that you have had. These could be things that have caused immense stress and have contributed in one way or another to your symptoms.

Note down all questions you have for your doctor.

So often, we have questions ready in our minds that we are planning to ask the doctor. Yet when we get there, we go completely blank. Prepare appropriately by writing down all possible questions to help make your appointment as informative as possible.

Some of the questions you can ask your doctor:

For your first appointment, include:

- What do you think is the cause of my condition and/or symptoms?
- What tests do you recommend that I take?
- Are there any lifestyle changes and forms of treatment that may help reduce and improve my symptoms?
- Do you recommend that I see a specialist?

For your appointment with a specialist:

Are there lifestyle changes I can make that can work without me having to take drugs?

What are the side effects I may experience from these drugs?

I have an underlying medical condition. What's the best way for me to manage them together?

Can I consume any alcohol during the treatment phase and even afterwards?

When should I expect to notice an improvement after starting my treatment?

Take a friend/ family member with you

It is possible that you can forget all the information a doctor shares with you during your appointment. Having a second person there will help you remember something you may have forgotten and give you moral support, especially when the doctor has some difficult information to process.

It is also important that you anticipate some of the questions that your doctor will ask you in your first and even subsequent appointments. Being prepared to provide answers will create a great environment to discuss in more detail issues that are of concern to you.

Some of the questions that your doctor may ask you include:

Take me through the symptoms you are experiencing.

When was the first time you experienced these symptoms?

Are your symptoms constant, or do they come and go?

Is there something that you have noticed that triggers these symptoms? Examples could be the food you eat, emotional or physical stress.

Do you suffer from any other medical condition that you are currently being treated for?

Does your immediate family have a history of gout?

Do you take alcohol? If you do, which type and how often?

Take me through what you eat on a normal day.

A Healthy You

We cannot downplay the tremendous impact that today's medicine has had on the health of the world's population. Through modern medicine, we have been able to successfully eradicate illnesses that wiped out entire communities in the past, such as the plague, malaria, and more.

However, it is also true that modern medicine primarily focuses on just treating the disease at hand and not the person.

Many of us are very familiar with popping pills for just about anything, whether a headache or cough. The problem with this is that we don't try to get to the root of the problem by questioning what is causing the headache or cough in the first place? Is it a way of your body trying to alert you of a deeper-rooted problem?

Your body is constantly sending you signals when there's a problem. The extreme fatigue you have been feeling without doing any intensive work is not something you dismiss by increasing your coffee or energy drink intake. Dry and itchy skin out of nowhere shouldn't be immediately treated with a soothing cream.

We must teach ourselves to listen to our bodies. Pay close attention to what is normal and what isn't and. This will enable you to immediately tell when something is wrong. If you have been diagnosed with gout, just think about the many times you went to your doctor with certain symptoms, and you were given medicine to treat those symptoms without further tests to determine if there was an underlying cause only after repeated flare-ups were tests done.

The domino effect

Consider the simple analogy of spraining your ankle. After spraining your ankle, it is normal to limp to shift weight from the injured leg. After days of limping, you start experiencing pain in your other foot. This is because it was forced to pick up the slack and is now carrying so much more weight than it is used to.

The same applies to other parts of your body. When something goes wrong in your body, it opens the door to other medical complications. For example, your diet is primarily made of refined food products, and you live a very dormant life. In time, you develop diabetes, and even then, it becomes very challenging for you to adjust your lifestyle. Slowly, your kidneys start taking the heat, and at your next health check-up, your doctor tells you that you've tested positive for kidney disease.

The point here is that you must make a conscious decision to take care of your body, starting with what goes into your digestive system, your mind and soul, and how you keep your body active. A holistic approach to life will help you realize that everything is interconnected, and you can help your body achieve good health again.

The Diet

If you eat food that nature has gifted you, without stripping it of any nutrients by refining it, then you are going to be the picture of health as you will be providing all of your organs with the nourishment they need. On the other hand, if you are always eating fast food, sugar, fat and salt-laden snacks, and a ton of soda, then your body is going to be filled with gunk which eventually presents as chronic illnesses.

What I am trying to say is that, generally by eating healthily, we are going to be healthy. Of course, there are unique situations where some of us are born with some medical conditions or have a genetic predisposition for a certain disease. But, even then, if we do our best to provide our bodies with the nutrition we need, then we are going to be the healthiest possible.

When it comes to gout, it is not a death sentence! With the right nutrition, you can lead a high quality of life for a very, very long time. The first thing about living healthy with gout, is you need to be very careful with what you eat. Limit the amount of food that is high in purines from your diet.

It's a mental game

Once you accept that you truly want to make a change in your life, it's normal to want to go cold turkey and replace most of the food you previously ate by cutting out all sugar and processed foods and hitting the gym hard from the onset. Sadly, this approach has a high failure rate.

To start with, you need to understand your body is naturally going to resist change no matter how beneficial it is. That is the basic survival DNA that is ingrained in us from the moment we are conceived. So, to work around this, prepare your mind by really thinking about what you stand to gain from embarking on a health journey. And to back this up, start with small and sustainable tweaks. You can start with a list of pros and cons to embarking on this journey.

Let healthy nutrition be the underlining factor.

You've heard it said that you are what you eat, and for you to achieve the best health, it's 80% nutrition and 20% fitness.

Take a picture or mental note of yourself and where you are before embarking on this new health journey, and then reflect on how you feel a month into it. Apart from noticing your clothes fitting a little loser, compare how your joints feel. Are you getting a gout flare-up? How long are the intervals between the attacks? How do you feel mentally and consider your general mood? Are you sleeping better? From my personal experience, you'll be kicking yourself for not having discovered this sooner!
Our healthy anti-inflammatory recipes will help flush out toxins from your body and provide the nutrition that your body actually needs, to relieve gout symptoms faster, especially when combined with a 30 minute daily or alternate-day workout.

Aim to eat only natural foods. Stay away from sugary carbonated drinks, fast food, and refined foods. As a rule of thumb, if it didn't come directly from a plant or animal, don't put it in your mouth.

Here is a list of foods that you should steer clear of:

- Sugary processed drinks: soda, concentrated juices
- French fries and potato chips
- Refined flour products: white bread, cookies, pastry
- Candy bars
- Some alcohol types such as beer
- Yeast-based foods
- Ice cream
- High-calorie milkshakes and smoothies

High- fructose foods – fructose which occurs in fruits and high fructose corn syrup often added to processed beverages and foods increase serum uric acid levels. Limiting intake of these foods or avoiding them altogether helps reduce the symptoms of gout or even prevent it.

The take-home message is the worst foods to eat when trying to lose weight are overly refined and processed foods. Read the labels to be sure of what you are eating. If you can't pronounce anything on the label, this is a sign you should not be eating it in the first place. Nature is perfectly equipped to provide us with the nutrition we need, so use it!

Listen to your body

Pay close attention to what your body is saying to you. For example, don't be too hard on yourself when cravings hit you when you are starting out. Look for low-fat and low-sugar alternatives that taste just as good and are actually good for you. It will take time for your body to accept your lifestyle change, and once it does, you will no longer be a prisoner to refined chocolate chip cookies. Instead, you will go for healthy almond chocolate cookies that are just as good, if not better!

You will soon find out which foods work for you and enjoy preparing them, knowing that you are taking care of yourself at the end of the day.

Who said that a healthy journey couldn't be fun?

Physical exercise

Our bodies were made to move. Dedicate a minimum of 30 minutes every day to this. It is vital that you find an exercise that you enjoy for you to be able to stick to it.

Working out gets your blood pumping to all organs, and it also helps eliminate toxins from the body through sweat which will go a long way in helping your kidneys in the process of uric acid elimination.

As a holistic approach, the exercise connects all of your organs and encourages them to work together in order to move in synchrony which is very important to your wellbeing.

When all of your organs feel needed and are put to the task, they work really well. It is, however, important to remember to stay safe to avoid injuries. If possible, take one day out of each week to exercise in the great outdoors. It could be anything from hiking up a mountain, cycling on a forest trail, or rowing a boat in a natural lake or ocean. Of course, this must be done in a controlled environment to ensure you are always safe.

Meditation

Meditation helps you detach from everything around you and to focus on only one thing. You can choose to shut off everything and concentrate on your mind, body, and soul connection. If you have never tried meditation, this may seem impossible. Start by going to a tranquil place which could even be within your house. If you have noisy neighbors, wear noise canceling headphones, sit very quiet, and try not to think of anything. With practice, you will find you can sit like this even for half an hour. This will bring profound calmness to your life and make your brain sharper, thus reducing stress in your life.

Your body is a temple, and if you take excellent care of it, you will enjoy the best quality of life. Before you put anything in your mouth, ask yourself whether it is fit for the temple. If it is, go ahead and enjoy, but if it's not, don't eat it. What may seem like just one bite of unhealthy food, when accumulated, could lead to serious problems in the future.

Practice mind, body, and soul health, and with time you will realize that you are able to make decisions that are only beneficial to your entire self. You will learn to tell when there's the slightest change in your body function. I can't say this enough; gout is not a death sentence! Now that you fully understand what it is all about and how you can tweak your lifestyle to slow or stop its progression, the ball is in your court!

Continue educating yourself more and others in need of this information.

Using Food to Reduce a Gout Attack

What you eat during a gout attack will either exacerbate or improve your symptoms. It would be best if you continued with a gout-healthy diet to reduce the duration of the attack. This is the time you should only eat foods that are very low in purines.

- **Foods containing high levels of vitamin C**

Vitamin C is rich in antioxidants, and it also plays an important role in lowering the amount of uric acid in the body. Vitamin C rich foods include oranges, grapefruit, lemon, lime, kale, spinach, sweet peppers, broccoli, strawberries, and tomatoes.

If you also have or are at a high risk of kidney stones, it's advisable to avoid vitamin C supplements.

A study that was first published in 2009 that followed approximately 47,000 adult males for the next 20 years regularly examined their risk of gout attacks and how this correlated to their intake of vitamin C. The researchers involved arrived at the conclusion that gout attacks were lowered by up to 45 percent when the patients took a minimum of 1500 mg of vitamin C every day.

- **Cherries**

Cherries are known for helping to treat urinary tract infections thanks to their anti-inflammatory and antioxidant properties. For the same reason, they have been studied for their role in managing and preventing gout.

They have been shown to lower uric acid levels in the body. Thanks to their antioxidant and anti-inflammatory properties, they decrease inflammation around joints, thus offering quick relief in the event of an attack and lowering the risk of future gout flare-ups.

Cherries can be consumed fresh, dried, or frozen, and because they are a natural food, there is no set amount that you should eat per day. You can add them to smoothies, a fruit or veggie salad, juice them or eat as is. A serving of a glass of natural cherry juice or half a serving of cherries is most common. When taking cherry supplements, follow the recommended serving size of the manufacturer.

The question of what type of cherry is most effective for preventing or reducing the risk of gout attacks has arisen. There are no clear results from research conducted that one type of cherry is better than the other between sweet cherries and tart cherries. The important thing is to buy organically grown cherries and make your own juice instead of buying processed cherry juice.

Coffee

Coffee is one of the highest consumed beverages globally, and it has been studied widely for its many health benefits. Some of the early studies concluded that coffee significantly reduced the risk of gout and gout flare-ups. However, more recent studies have shown that these benefits vary based on gender.

A study conducted in 2015 that reviewed earlier studies showed that the risk of gout was reduced by 40 percent in males who took at least 4 cups of coffee every day while those who drank a minimum of 6 cups of coffee a day reduced their risk of gout by 59 percent.

The same study indicated that women who drank a minimum of 1 cup of coffee and up to 3 cups of coffee a day reduced their risk of gout by 22 percent and those who took more than four cups of coffee in a day reduced their risk by up to 57 percent.

The researchers' conclusion was that drinking four cups of coffee a day for both males and females lowered the levels of uric acid in the body, therein reducing the risk of gout.

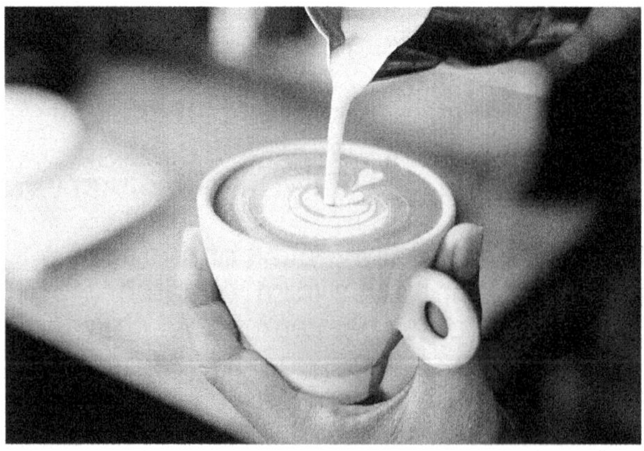

Low-purine foods

The most obvious way to reduce your risk of gout is to consume low purine foods. One such diet is the dash diet which is mostly followed by people suffering from inflammation. It features low-purine foods that are extremely beneficial to people who are at a high risk of gout.

Foods that are low in purines include those we have mentioned already, such as cherries, citrus fruits, and others such as plant-based high protein foods like veggies, legumes, seeds, and nuts, and also low-fat dairy foods.

Water

This natural ingredient has tons of health benefits. For people predisposed to getting gout or already have it, drinking a lot of water helps in the excretion of uric acid.

Recipes for Success

We are now moving to the food section. Check out our sweet and savory collection of recipes that will help prevent and reduce gout symptoms. Here, you will find the tastiest and healthiest meals, snacks, and drinks that are anything but boring!

Purines food list

High: 150-1,000mg purine per 100g

Wild or farmed game: Venison, Rabbit/Hare, Pheasant, Quail, Grouse.

Organ meat: Pate, Terrine, Liver, Kidneys, Heart.

Extracts of Meat and Yeast: Bovril, Oxo, Marmite, Vegemite

Fish Roe: Caviar, Taramasalata.

Some Seafood: Scallops, Herrings, Mackerel, Trout, Crayfish, Lobster, Tuna,

Redfish and Carp

Small Fish – Whole or Processed: Anchovies, Sardines, Sprats, Whitebait and Anchovy paste.

Moderate: 50-150mg purine per 100g

Poultry: Duck, Turkey, Goose, and Chicken.

Red Meats and Sausages: Beef, Lamb, Pork, Bacon, Ham, and Veal.

Fish and Seafood: Mussels, Prawns, Oysters, and Most Other Shellfish, Shrimp,

Scampi, Plaice, Cod, Haddock, Pike-perch, Salmon.

Lentils, Peas and Beans, Chickpeas, Hummus, Soya Beans, Bean Curd, Tofu,

Tempeh and Miso

Peanuts, Cashews and Ground Nuts

Cauliflower, Kale, Brussel sprouts, Broccoli/Calabrese, Chinese greens, Leek,

Asparagus, Spinach, and Mushrooms

Low : 0-50mg purine per 100g

Vegetables: All are fine (except those in the moderate group)

Green beans, French beans, Sugar snap peas, Sweet corn, Beetroot, Carrot, Cucumber, Fennel, Lettuce, Potato, Pumpkin, Quince, Radishes, Rhubarb, Summer Squash, and Onion

Dairy Products: Milk, creams, yogurt, ice cream, cheese, and eggs

Nuts: Most nuts (except peanuts or cashews; they are moderate).

High Fructose Food.

These can be eaten but in moderaton:

Apples, Grapes, Lychees, Mangos, Pears, Prunes, Watermelon, Dried fruits.

Tomatoes, Broccoli, Cauliflower, Corn, Sweet potato, Green beans, Green peas, Green peppers.

Tomato sauces, Sweetcorn, Sugar snap peas and pickles

Agave syrup, Caramel Fructose, Corn Syrup, Honey, Invert Sugar Licorice, Molasses, Pancake Syrup, Palm Sugar

Fun Facts

Tomatoes and Gout

Traditionally tomatoes have been considered to be a gout-friendly food. However, some recent studies have shown it to trigger gout in some people. Although tomatoes are low in purines, research has found about 20 percent of people with gout report tomatoes may be the trigger.

It is worth remembering that your genetics and overall health can make a more significant difference in how foods such as tomatoes trigger gout. This means tomatoes may cause a gout flare-up in one person but do not cause any reaction in another.

Tomatoes are nutrient-rich and high in vitamin C.

If you feel tomatoes are triggering your gout flare-up, try substituting it with something else like squash, bell peppers, eggplant.

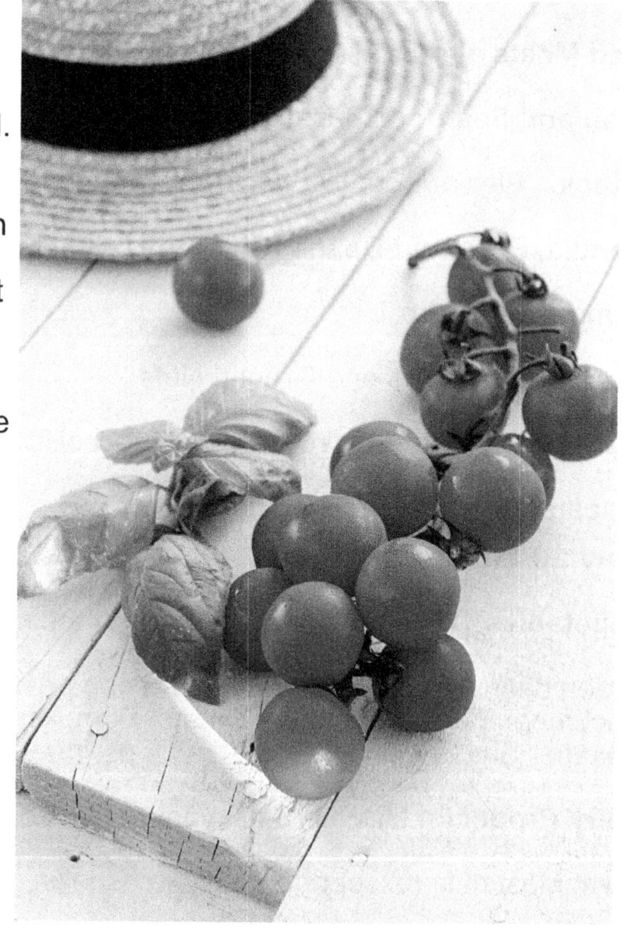

Coriander

Coriander/cilantro is widely being used to reduce creatine and uric acid in the blood. The leaves can help accelerate the normalization of the uric acid and creatinine levels along with your medication. Coriander is also good for urine flow.

It may also help lower your blood sugar, fight infections, and is good for your heart, brain, skin, and digestive health.

Pack with vitamins and minerals like Vitamin A, Vitamin C, Vitamin K, Iron, and Calcium.

Turmeric

Many studies show that turmeric has significant benefits for your body and brain. Most of these benefits come from its main active ingredient, curcumin.

Curcumin is known to be a powerful anti-inflammatory and antioxidant. Scientists believe that chronic low-level inflammation can play a role in some health conditions and diseases.

- cancer
- metabolic syndrome
- Alzheimer's disease
- heart disease

It is believed that curcumin suppresses many molecules known to play major roles in inflammation. That's why anything that can help fight chronic inflammation is a potentially important tool in preventing and helping treat these conditions.

Many brain disorders are linked to decreased BDNF proteins, like depression and Alzheimer's disease. There have now been significant studies to show that curcumin may actually boost the levels of BDNF in the brain.

Doing this may effectively delay or even reverse many brain diseases, including age-related decreases in brain function. Although, since these studies were performed on animals, it's hard to say what the results mean for humans.

None the less it seems turmeric is a powerful spice indeed.

Breakfast
AND BRUNCH

"Begin the day with a positive mindset, and you will have a beautiful day!".

Jade Patterson

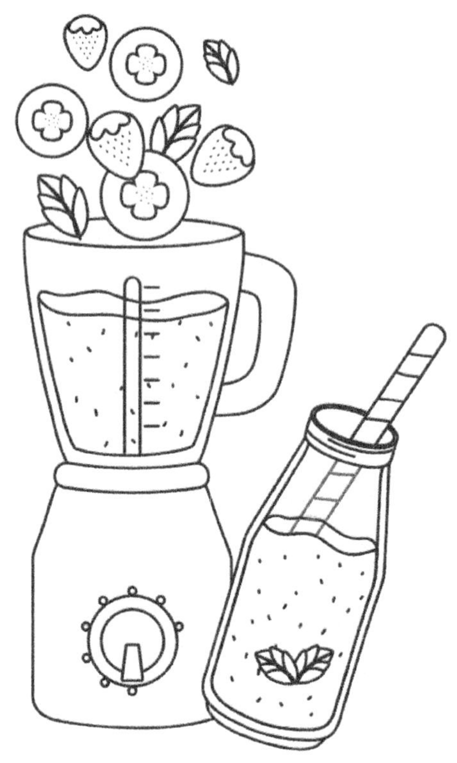

Healthy Nutty Breakfast Muesli

Yield: 24 Servings of ¼ cup each
Total Time: 5 Minutes
Prep Time: 5 Minutes
Cook Time: N/A

Ingredients
3 cups rolled oats
¼ cup hemp seeds
½ cup chia seeds
½ cup pumpkin seeds
½ cup sunflower seeds
¼ cup dried apricot
½ cup dried bananas chips, chopped
¼ cup chopped hazelnut
¼ cup chopped almonds
½ cup unsweetened toasted coconut flakes

Directions
Mix seeds, dry fruit, and toasted coconut flakes in a large bowl; stir until well combined. Then place the mixture in a large airtight container for storage.

Serve topped with milk and fresh berries.

Stored in an airtight container, this has a shelf life of 4 weeks.

Nutritional Information per Serving:
Calories: 89; Total Fat: 5g; Net Carbs: 7.6g; Dietary Fiber: 2.2g; Sugars: 2.2g; Protein: 3g; Sodium: 10.7 mg

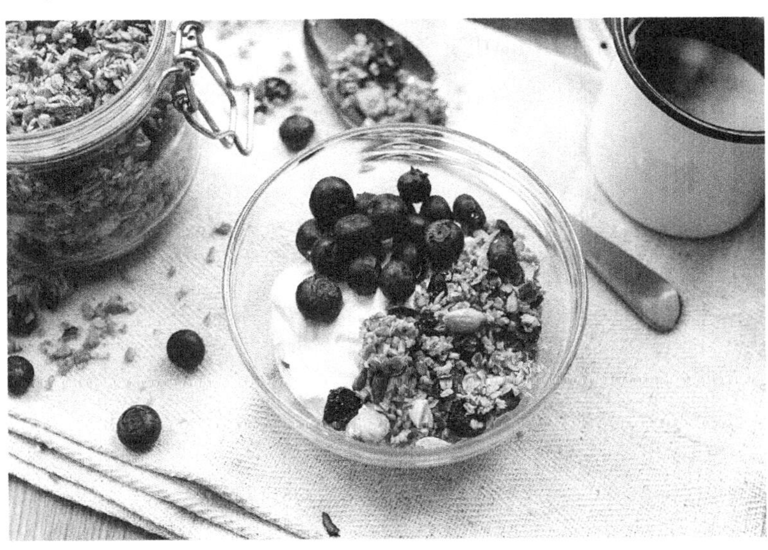

Citrus Avocado Superfood Detox Smoothie Bowl

Yield: 3 Servings
Total Time: 5 Minutes
Prep Time: 5 Minutes
Cook Time: N/A

Ingredients
1 avocado
2 banana
1 cup low-fat plain yogurt
2 cups unsweetened almond milk
1 tablespoon lemon juice
1 orange
1 grapefruit
1 cup blueberries
2 cup baby spinach
1 teaspoon chia seeds
¼ cup toasted chopped walnuts

Directions
Blend all ingredients until very smooth apart from the seeds and nuts. Serve with a sprinkling of chia seeds and chopped walnuts on top.

Nutritional Info per Serving:
Calories: 365; Total Fat: 15g; Carbs: 42.3g; Dietary Fiber: 10g; Sugars: 21g; Protein: 19.9g; Sodium: 260mg

Detoxifying Tropical Fruit Smoothie Breakfast Bowls

Yield: 3 Servings
Total Time: 5 Minutes
Prep Time: 5 Minutes
Cook Time: N/A

Ingredients

1 cup chopped fresh pineapple
1 medium banana, frozen
2 cups frozen mango, diced
½ freshly squeezed lemon juice
3 cups light coconut milk
¼ cup toasted coconut flakes
¼ cup chopped almond nuts

Directions

Blend banana, mango, lemon juice, pineapple, coconut milk until smooth in a blender.

Divide the mixture among serving bowls; top each serving with toasted coconut and chopped almonds.

Nutritional Information per Serving:

Calories: 341; Total Fat: 14g; Carbs: 31g; Dietary Fiber: 3.3g; Sugars: 32g; Protein: 5g; Sodium: 84mg

Antioxidant-Rich Citrus Avocado & Blackberry Smoothie Bowl with Toasted Nuts

Yield: 4 Servings
Total Time: 5 Minutes
Prep Time: 5 Minutes
Cook Time: N/A

Ingredients
2 cups fresh blackberries
1 cup fresh raspberries
2 cups fresh spinach
3 cups unsweetened almond milk
½ grapefruit, peeled, segmented
½ cup fresh lemon juice
1 avocado
2 bananas
2 tablespoons toasted pumpkin seeds
½ cup toasted coconut flakes
½ cup toasted chopped almonds

Directions
Blend the berries, almond milk, avocado, lemon juice, grapefruit, bananas, and spinach until smooth and creamy in a blender.

Divide the smoothie among serving bowls and top each serving with freshly toasted almonds, pumpkin seeds, and toasted coconut flakes.

Nutritional Information per Serving:
Calories: 290; Total Fat: 16.3g; Net Carbs: 37g; Dietary Fiber: 11g; Sugars: 18g; Protein: 6.3g; Sodium: 162mg

Almond & Berry Breakfast Smoothie

Yield: 2 Servings
Total Time: 5 Minutes
Prep Time: 5 Minutes
Cook Time: N/A

Ingredients

½ cup blackberries
½ cup blueberries
½ cup raspberries
½ cup strawberries
3 cups unsweetened almond milk
1 avocado
½ teaspoon cinnamon
½ teaspoon liquid stevia
2 tablespoons almond butter
½ cup plain low-fat yogurt

Directions

Blend everything together until very smooth.

Nutritional Information per Serving:

Calories: 344; Total Fat: 24.1g; Net Carbs: 24.9g; Dietary Fiber: 10.6g; Sugars: 12g; Protein: 10g; Sodium: 315mg

Anti-Inflammatory Avocado & Blueberry Smoothie

Yield: 3 Servings
Total Time: 5 Minutes
Prep Time: 5 Minutes
Cook Time: N/A

Ingredients
3 cups unsweetened almond milk
1 avocado, diced
2 banana's
1 tablespoon chia seeds
1 tablespoon almond butter
1 teaspoon minced fresh ginger
2 tablespoons of lemon juice
1 tablespoons lemon zest
1 cup frozen blueberries
2 tablespoons toasted coconut flakes
1 teaspoon liquid stevia

Directions
Combine all ingredients in a blender and blend until smooth and creamy.

Divide the smoothie between serving bowls and top each with more blueberries and coconut flakes.

Nutrition information per Serving:
Calories: 341; Total Fat: 7.4g; Net Carbs: 39.1g; Dietary Fiber: 9.7g; Sugars: 18.6g; Protein: 7.4g; Sodium: 202mg

Pineapple & Ginger Detox Smoothie

Yield: 2 Servings
Total Time: 5 Minutes
Prep Time: 5 Minutes
Cook Time: N/A

Ingredients
2 cups pineapple chunks
1 teaspoon ginger, minced
½ teaspoon ground turmeric
2 tablespoons lemon juice
1 tablespoon of chia seeds
1 banana
1 ½ cups coconut water

Directions
Combine all the ingredients in your blender and pulse until smooth.

Serve in a tall glass.

Nutritional Information per Serving:
Calories: 157; Total Fat: 2.7g; Carbs: 33.7g; Dietary Fiber 7g; Sugars: 14.4g; Protein: 3g; Sodium: 164mg

Chai-Almond Green Smoothie

Yield: 2 Servings
Total Time: 5 Minutes
Prep Time: 5 Minutes
Cook Time: N/A

Ingredients
2 cups unsweetened almond milk
1 banana
1 tablespoon of chia seeds
1 cup of kale
1 cup of spinach
2 tablespoons almond butter
¼ teaspoon ground nutmeg
¼ teaspoon ground cardamom
½ teaspoon ground cinnamon
½ teaspoon ground ginger
½ teaspoon vanilla extract

Directions
Blend all the ingredients until very smooth.

Serve in a tall glass.

Nutritional Information per Serving:
Calories: 250; Total Fat: 14g; Carbs: 26g; Dietary Fiber: 8g; Sugars: 8.9g; Protein: 12g; Sodium: 260mg

Overnight Oats Fruit ‘n’ Nut Breakfast Smoothie

Yield: 2 Servings
Total Time: 10 Minutes
Prep Time: 10 Minutes
Cook Time: N/A

Ingredients
2 tablespoons almond butter
1 ½ cups unsweetened almond milk
½ cup of oats
1 banana
½ cup pitted dates, chopped
1 teaspoon of hemp seeds
1 tablespoon of chia seeds
2 tablespoons toasted chopped almonds for topping

Directions
Place all the ingredients apart from the almonds in a medium bowl and pour over the almond milk. Cover the bowl with cling wrap and chill in the fridge overnight.

Combine all the ingredients, apart from the chopped almonds in your blender, and pulse until you achieve your desired consistency.

Serve in a tall glass and top with the chopped almonds.

Nutritional Information per Serving:
Calories: 330; Total Fat: 16g; Carbs: 39g; Dietary Fiber: 8.5g; Sugars: 23g; Protein: 9g; Sodium: 148mg

Healthy Omelet with Lemony Avocado-Tomato Salsa

Yields: 3 Servings
Total Time: 40 Minutes
Prep Time: 10 Minutes
Cook Time: 30 Minutes

Ingredients
1 red onion, chopped
2 cloves garlic, minced
6 large free-range eggs, beaten
2 tablespoons fresh lemon juice
1 teaspoon of lemon zest
1 medium avocado, diced
2 medium tomatoes, diced
3 spring onions, chopped
1 tablespoon coconut oil
Pinch salt and black pepper
1 tablespoon chopped coriander

Directions
In a small bowl, toss together fresh lemon juice, lemon zest, avocado, tomato, spring onions, and coriander; season with sea salt and pepper and set aside.

In a separate bowl, beat the eggs and set them aside.

Set a frying pan over medium heat; add coconut oil and heat until hot. Sauté red onions and garlic until fragrant. Then set aside.

Add a third of the egg mixture to the pan and tilt to cover the bottom of the pan. Cook for about 2 minutes per side and then transfer to a plate.

Repeat with the remaining ingredients for the second and third omelet. Serve the omelet topped with the avocado-tomato mixture and sauté onions/garlic.

Nutritional Information per Serving:
Calories: 327; Total Fat: 33g; Net Carbs: 15g; Dietary Fiber: 4.6g; Sugars: 3.1g; Protein: 16.4 g; Sodium: 70mg

Spiced Omelet with Red Onions & Chili

Yield: 2 Servings
Total Time: 15 Minutes
Prep Time: 5 Minutes
Cook Time: 10 Minutes

Ingredients
2 tablespoons olive oil
1 red onion, chopped
1 green chili, chopped seeds removed
2 tomatoes, chopped
¼ teaspoon chili powder
4 eggs
4 tablespoons milk
1 teaspoon lemon juice
½ teaspoon turmeric powder
2 tablespoons coriander/cilantro, chopped
1 teaspoon fresh thyme
Pinch salt and pepper

Directions
In a bowl, combine fresh thyme, chili powder, coriander, green chili, tomatoes, chopped onions, and turmeric powder until well blended; whisk in the eggs, milk, and season with salt and pepper.

In a frying pan, heat oil and then pour in about half of the mixture; swirl the pan to spread the egg mixture and cook for about 2 minutes per side or until the egg is set. Sprinkle with lemon juice and some fresh coriander. Transfer to a plate and keep warm.

Repeat with the remaining mixture. Serve hot with a glass of fresh orange juice or hot coffee for a satisfying breakfast.

Nutritional Infomation per Serving:
Calories: 239; Total Fat: 23.4g; Net Carbs: 14g; Dietary Fiber: 2.3 g; Sugars: 5g; Protein: 16g; Sodium: 123mg

Mango, Pineapple & Beet Chia Pudding Parfait with Toasted Nuts

Yield: 4 Servings
Total Time: 10 Minutes
Prep Time: 10 Minutes
Chill Time: Overnight

Ingredients

½ cup chia seeds
½ teaspoon liquid stevia
1 teaspoon vanilla extract
1 ½ cups unsweetened almond milk
1 teaspoon matcha green tea powder
3 tablespoons fresh beetroot juice
1 whole mango
1 cup of pineapple chunks
½ fresh lemon, juiced
1 tablespoon of fresh ginger
½ cup toasted almonds, chopped
¼ pistachio nuts, chopped

Directions

In 2 small bowls, evenly split the almond milk, chia seeds, liquid stevia, and vanilla extract. In one bowl, add the green tea powder, and in the other, add the beetroot and ginger. Mix both bowls well. Cover and refrigerate overnight. The following day stir both mixtures well.

In a food processor, puree the fresh mango, pineapple, and lemon juice until fine.

To assemble, layer the green tea chia pudding in the bottom of serving glasses, followed by the pureed mango and then the beetroot layer. Top with toasted nuts for a crunchy finish.

Nutritional Information per Serving:

Calories: 253; Total Fat: 12.1g; Carbs: 25g; Dietary Fiber: 14g; Sugars: 10.3g; Protein: 8.8g; Sodium: 84mg

Smoked Salmon Frittata

Yield: 4 servings
Total Time: 30 Minutes
Prep Time: 10 Minutes
Cook Time: 20 Minutes

Ingredients
2 tablespoons extra-virgin olive oil
1 red onion, chopped
6 spring onions, trimmed and chopped
200g smoked salmon, sliced into small pieces
8 large eggs
3 tablespoons chopped dill
2 tablespoons thyme
120g light cheddar cheese
2 tablespoons light sour cream
Pinch salt and black pepper

Directions
Preheat your oven to 350°F/ 177°C
Place a large ovenproof pan over medium heat; add oil and heat until hot. Stir in onions and sauté, stirring, for about 4 minutes or until tender and soft.

Beat the eggs, spring onions, dill, thyme, sour cream, and cheese in a bowl. Season with salt and black pepper, then pour into the pan.

Arrange the salmon onto the egg mixture.

Cook for 8 minutes or until almost set.

Transfer to the oven and cook until golden.

Remove the frittata from the oven and transfer to a serving plate; slice and serve with a glass of freshly squeezed orange juice or a hot coffee.

Nutritional Information per Serving:
Calories: 378; Total Fat: 25g; Net Carbs: 7.7g; Dietary Fiber: 1.2; Sugars: 1.7g; Protein: 31g; Sodium: 409mg

Lemon Raspberry Pancakes

Yield: 4 Servings
Total Time: 15 Minutes
Prep Time: 5 Minutes
Cook Time: 10 Minutes

Ingredients
1 cup almond flour
¼ cup coconut flour
½ teaspoon baking soda
Pinch salt
¾ cup unsweetened almond milk
3 free-range eggs
1 tablespoon maple syrup
2 tablespoon coconut oil
1 teaspoon vanilla extract
1 teaspoon lemon zest
2 tablespoons fresh lemon juice
1 cup fresh raspberries

Directions
In a large bowl, whisk together eggs, vanilla, maple syrup, and lemon zest until well combined; whisk in coconut flour until well blended. Whisk in almond flour, baking soda, salt, and lemon juice until very smooth.

Heat coconut oil in a frying pan set over medium heat; add in two spoonfuls of the batter and spread into a circle. Cook for about 2 minutes per side and then repeat with the remaining ingredients. Divide the fresh raspberries among the pancakes. Serve warm.

Nutritional Information per Serving:
Calories: 300; Total Fat: 18g; Net Carbs: 21g; Dietary Fiber: 10.7g; Sugars: 4.5g; Protein: 13g; Sodium: 232mg

Healthy Detox Grain-Free Porridge

Yield: 1 Serving
Total Time: 7 Minutes
Prep Time: 2 Minutes
Cook Time: 5 Minutes

Ingredients
½ cup unsweetened almond milk
2 tablespoons flaxseed meal
1 tablespoon hemp seeds
2 tablespoon chia seeds
¼ teaspoon cinnamon powder
1 tablespoon toasted coconut flakes
1 tablespoon toasted almonds,
3 dried apricots, chopped

Directions
Warm the almond milk and cinnamon on a stovetop for a few minutes. Do not allow it to boil over. In a bowl, mix the flaxseeds, hemp seeds, chia seeds, apricots; pour the warm milk over the seed mix. Allow it to sit for a minute, then top with toasted coconut flakes and almonds.

Nutritional Information per Serving:
Calories: 335; Total Fat: 30g; Net Carbs: 27g; Dietary Fiber: 9 g; Sugars: 17g; Protein: 13g; Sodium: 129mg

Healthy Tropical Fruit Parfaits with Nut Whip Topping

Yield: 4 Servings
Total Time: 15 Minutes
Prep Time: 15 Minutes
Cook Time: N/A

Ingredients
Nut Whip Topping
6 dates pitted and soaked
¾ cup cashews, soaked and drained
3 tbsp softened coconut cream
Tropical Fruit Parfaits
2 kiwis and thinly sliced
1 mango, peeled and diced
2 bananas, sliced
1 cup of strawberries chopped
1 orange, juiced
2 tablespoons toasted coconut flakes

Directions
In a blender, combine the coconut cream, cashew nuts, and dates; blend until smooth. Chill the topping for at least 1 hour before serving.

In a bowl, combine all the diced parfait ingredients with the orange juice and mix well.

In serving glasses, layer the parfait mixture and top with the nut topping; repeat the layers to fill the glasses.

Top each with toasted coconut flakes and serve chilled.

Nutritional Information per Serving:
Calories: 344; Total Fat: 17.25g; Carbs: 48g; Dietary Fiber: 5.7g; Sugars: 30g; Protein: 8.25g; Sodium: 58mg

Delicious Gluten-Free Avocado Pancakes

Yield: 4 Servings
Total Time: 15 Minutes
Prep Time: 5 Minutes
Cook Time: 10 Minutes

Ingredients
1 ripe avocado
2 cups almond flour
¼ cup tapioca flour
2 eggs
1 tablespoon fresh lemon juice and zest
1 teaspoon honey
¾ cup unsweetened almond milk
1 teaspoon baking powder
1 teaspoon matcha powder
1 teaspoon vanilla extract
Pinch of salt
1 cup fresh berries to serve

Directions
In a blender, blend together the avocado, lemon juice, lemon zest, honey, vanilla, almond milk until nice and smooth.

Then mix together almond flour, tapioca flour, salt, matcha powder, and the baking powder. Transfer the avocado mixture and fold it into the flour mixture. Mix until well combined.

Heat oil in a frying pan over medium heat; add in batter and spread into a circle.

Cook for approximately 2 to 3 minutes per side or until browned. Repeat with the remaining batter.
Serve topped with fresh berries for your choice

Nutritional Information per Serving:
Calories: 389; Total Fat: 28g; Net Carbs: 20g; Dietary Fiber: 8.5g; Sugars: 3g; Protein: 12.5g; Sodium: 83.3mg

Spiced Scrambled Eggs

Yield: 2 Serving
Total Time: 15 Minutes
Prep Time: 5 Minutes
Cook Time: 10 Minutes

Ingredients
1 tablespoon extra-virgin olive oil
½ red onion, diced
½ bell pepper, diced
¼ teaspoon thyme
4 free-range eggs
¼ teaspoon red pepper flakes
¼ teaspoon cumin
1 tomato, chopped
Pinch of sea salt and pepper

Directions
Heat oil in a nonstick frying pan set over medium heat; stir in red onion and diced bell pepper and sauté for about 4 minutes or until onions are soft.

Meanwhile, in a bowl, whisk together eggs, thyme, red pepper flakes, salt and pepper, and cumin until frothy; add to onion mixture and cook, stirring slowly, until eggs are set.

Stir in chopped tomato and season with salt and pepper, and serve with toast.

Nutrition Information per Serving:
Calories: 261; Total Fat: 30g; Carbs: 8.5g; Dietary Fiber: 1g; Sodium: 80mg
Protein: 15.8g ; Sugars: 2.5g

Breakfast Guacamole with Whole-Wheat Bread

Yield: 6 Servings
Total Time: 10 Minutes
Prep Time: 10 Minutes
Cook Time: N/A

Ingredients
2 medium avocadoes
2 tablespoons chopped sun-dried tomatoes
10 cherry tomatoes, halved
2 tablespoons freshly squeezed lemon juice
½ red onion, finely chopped
A handful of freshly chopped cilantro/coriander
1 teaspoon fresh oregano, chopped
Pinch sea salt
½ teaspoon black pepper
6 slices of whole-wheat bread

Directions
Cut the avocadoes in half and remove the seed. Scoop out the flesh into a large bowl and use a fork to mash it up to desired consistency.

Sprinkle the lemon juice on the mashed avocado and mix well until combined. Add in all the remaining ingredients and mix well until well incorporated.

Adjust the salt, pepper, and herbs, if need be. If you like your guacamole more tangy, squeeze in more lemon juice and add the sun-dried tomatoes for a stronger tomato flavor.

Serve immediately with whole-wheat bread.

Nutritional Information per Serving:
Calories: 167; Total Fat: 10.8g; Net Carbs: 18.2g; Dietary Fiber: 4.9g; Sugars: 2.2g; Protein: 4.6g; Sodium: 168.5mg

Spiced Fried Egg and Avocado Toast

Yield: 1 Serving
Total Time: 5 Minutes
Prep Time: 5 Minutes
Cook Time: N/A

Ingredients
1 slice toasted whole wheat bread
1 fried egg
½ tomato, sliced
¼ ripe avocado, sliced
A pinch of parsley
A pinch of red pepper flakes
A pinch of salt and pepper

Directions
Spread the whole-wheat toast with mashed avocado and top with the fried egg and sliced tomato.

Sprinkle with red pepper flakes, parsley, salt, and pepper; serve right away.

Nutritional Information per Serving:
Calories: 161; Total Fat: 7g; Net Carbs: 19g; Dietary Fiber: 7g; Sugars: 3g; Protein: 5g; Sodium: 265mg

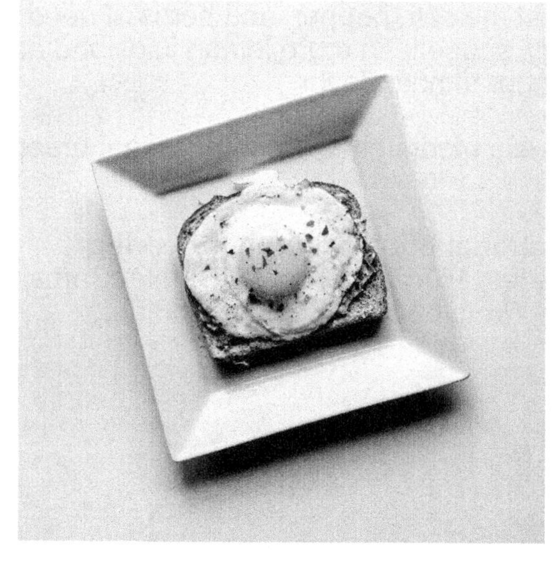

Superfood Cherry and Pineapple Overnight Oats

Yield: 2 Servings
Total Time: 10 Minutes
Chilling Time: Overnight
Prep Time: 10 Minutes
Cook Time: N/A

Ingredients
1 cup old-fashioned oats
1 teaspoon chia seeds
1 teaspoon hemp seeds
½ cup cherries, pitted and chopped
¾ cup vanilla almond milk (unsweetened)
¼ cup chopped fresh pineapple
¼ cup nonfat Greek yogurt
¼ teaspoon cinnamon
2 tablespoon chopped toasted almonds

Directions
Combine oats, chia seeds, hemp seeds, almond milk, cherries, pineapple, yogurt, cinnamon, and chopped toasted almonds, cover in a small bowl, and refrigerate overnight.

To serve, remove from the fridge and stir to mix well before serving

Nutritional Information per Serving:
Calories: 250; Total Fat: 9g; Net Carbs: 28g; Dietary Fiber: 6g; Sugars: 11g
Protein: 12.5g; Sodium: 114mg

Coconut Buckwheat Pancakes

Yield: 4 Servings
Total Time: 35 Minutes
Prep Time: 10 Minutes
Cook Time: 15 Minutes

Ingredients
½ cup coconut flour
½ cup buckwheat flour
1 teaspoon baking powder
⅛ teaspoon ground cinnamon
½ teaspoon salt
1 tablespoon sugar
½ teaspoon pure vanilla extract
1 ¼ cups low-fat coconut milk
2 eggs, beaten
2 tablespoons oil

Directions
In a large bowl, mix together all the dry ingredients.

In another bowl, whisk together wet ingredients, then pour into the buckwheat flour mixture and mix well.

Grease a non-stick frying pan with a bit of oil. Using a ¼-cup measure, scoop the batter onto the warm pan, cook for about 2 to 3 minutes per side.

Repeat with the remaining batter.

Serve with berries of your choice and a glass of orange juice.

Nutritional Information per Serving:
Calories: 262; Total Fat: 12g; Net Carbs: 32g; Dietary Fiber: 8.1g; Sugars: 4.5g Protein: 9g; Sodium: 186mg

Chai-Almond Latte Oatmeal with Banana and Apple

Yield: 4 Servings
Total Time: 30 Minutes
Prep Time: 10 Minutes
Cook Time: 20 Minutes

Ingredients
2 cups low-fat coconut creamer
4 Chai tea bags
2 cups unsweetened almond milk
1 ½ cups oats
½ teaspoon cinnamon
2 tablespoons toasted coconut
½ cup almonds chopped
2 bananas, sliced
1 apple diced
½ teaspoon sea salt

Directions
Simmer a cup of low-fat coconut creamer in a small saucepan over medium heat; add the tea bags and ¼ teaspoon of cinnamon; steep for about 10 minutes.

In the meantime, simmer the remaining coconut creamer and almond milk over medium to low heat, then stir in the oats; simmer for about 15 minutes or until thick.

Stir in strained chai cream and sea salt; ladle into serving bowls and top with toasted coconut, chopped almonds, diced apple, sliced banana, and more cinnamon.

Nutritional Information per Serving:
Calories: 292 Total Fat: 12g; Carbs: 41g; Dietary Fiber: 5.4g; Sugars: 22g; Protein: 4.9g; Sodium: 398mg

Spicy Breakfast Carrot Pudding

Yield: 4 Servings
Total Time: 45 Minutes
Prep Time: 10 Minutes
Cook Time: 15 Minutes
Chill Time: 20 Minutes

Ingredients

1 cup light coconut milk
1 ½ cups unsweetened almond milk
2 cup shredded carrots
3 tablespoons of chopped almonds
¼ teaspoon ground cloves
½ teaspoon ground cinnamon
½ teaspoon ground ginger
¼ teaspoon ground cardamom
¼ teaspoon ground turmeric
½ teaspoon liquid stevia
2 bananas sliced

Directions

In a saucepan set over medium heat, combine ½ cup coconut milk, ½ cup almond milk, and shredded carrots. Then stir in ginger, cardamom, turmeric, and cloves cooking for about 15 minutes or until tender carrots. Remove from heat and set aside to cool.

Transfer the carrots along with cooking liquid to a blender and pulse until just smooth.

Add stevia and the remaining milk and continue pulsing until combined.

Refrigerate for about 15 minutes or until set. Serve into serving bowls topped with sliced banana, chopped almonds, and a sprinkle of cinnamon.

Nutritional Information per Serving:
Calories: 164; Total Fat: 6.5g; Carbs: 23.2g; Dietary Fiber: 4.5g; Sugars: 11g; Protein: 3.75g; Sodium: 127mg

Chia Pudding with Toasted Coconut & Cherries

Yield: 2 Servings
Total Time: 45 Minutes
Prep Time: 10 Minutes
Chill Time: 30 Minutes or Overnight

Ingredients

6 tablespoons chia seeds
2 cups light coconut milk
½ teaspoon liquid stevia
¼ teaspoon spirulina powder
1 ripe banana
½ cup cherries pitted
2 tablespoons toasted coconut flakes

Directions

In a bowl, mix chia seeds, stevia, and half of the coconut milk; let it sit for at least 30 minutes or until all liquid is absorbed.

In a food processor, blend the remaining coconut milk, spirulina, and banana, until smooth.

Divide the chia seed mixture into serving jars and top each serving with a layer of spirulina puree. Serve topped with toasted coconut flakes and cherries.

Nutritional Information per Serving:

Calories: 416; Total Fat: 25.4g; Net Carbs: 41.4g; Dietary Fiber: 19.4g; Sugars: 13g; Protein: 13.4g; Sodium: 58mg

Christmas Spiced Pancakes

Yield: 4 Servings
Total Time: 25 Minutes
Prep Time: 10 Minutes
Cook Time: 15 Minutes

Ingredients
2 tablespoons coconut oil
1 cup light coconut milk
1 ¼ cup all-purpose flour
1 ½ teaspoons of baking powder
1 egg
1 tablespoon maple syrup
½ teaspoon salt
¼ teaspoon ground ginger
1 teaspoon ground cinnamon
½ teaspoon nutmeg
¼ teaspoon ground cloves

Directions
In a large bowl, mix together all the dry ingredients. In another bowl, whisk together the egg and all wet ingredients. Then pour the wet ingredients into the flour bowl; mix well until smooth.

Melt the oil in a frying pan over low to medium heat

Then add approximately ¼ cup of batter to the pan.

Cook for about 2 to 3 minutes per side or until golden. Transfer to a plate and keep warm; repeat with the remaining batter and oil.

Serve the pancakes with freshly made green tea or orange juice.

Nutritional Information per Serving:
Calories: 195; Total Fat: 4.9g; Carbs: 28g; Dietary Fiber: 2.5g; Sugars: 2g; Protein: 5.5g; Sodium: 324mg

Lunch

AND LIGHT MEALS

"The adventure starts with one single step.
Take that step, and the journey will begin.."

Jade Patterson

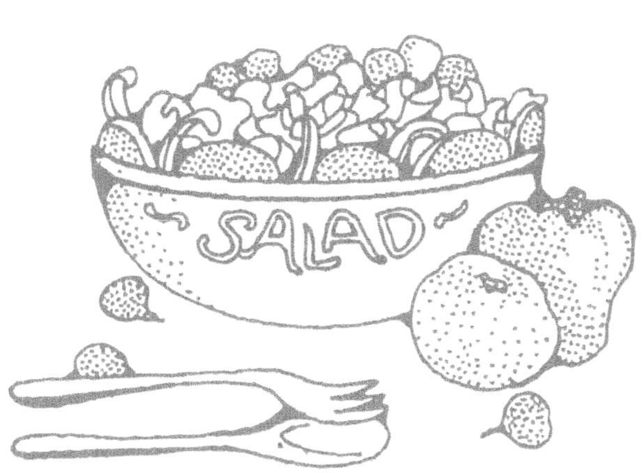

Spicy Mushroom Soup with Caramelized Red Onions

Yield: 3 Servings
Total Time: 20 Minutes
Prep Time: 10 Minutes
Cook Time: 10 Minutes

Ingredients

3 tablespoons extra-virgin olive oil
500g mushroom, trimmed
3 clove garlic, minced
3 Bay leaves
1 tsp smoked paprika
½ teaspoon chili flakes
½ teaspoon minced ginger
1 red onions, chopped
4 cups vegetable stock
1 tablespoon fresh thyme
½ teaspoon sea salt
Thyme sprigs
1 teaspoon black pepper
1 lemon, juiced and zest
1 spring onions, chopped

Directions

Fry the mushrooms, garlic, and one diced onion in oil and lemon juice until tender; set aside.

In a soup pot, sauté the second red diced onion in extra-virgin olive oil for about 5 minutes or until caramelized. Stir in vegetable stock, bay leaves, and spices; cook for a few minutes.

Place half of the caramelized onions and half of the mushroom in a blender; blend until very smooth; add garlic and thyme, and continue mixing until smooth and creamy.

Return the blended mushrooms to the soup pot and season with salt, thyme sprigs, and pepper.

Remove from heat and stir in fresh lemon juice and zest. To serve, top with the remaining mushrooms, spring onions and caramelized onions!

Nutritional Information per Serving:

Calories: 170; Total Fat: 10.3g; Net Carbs: 15g; Dietary Fiber: 3g; Sugars: 4g; Protein: 7.3g; Sodium: 930mg

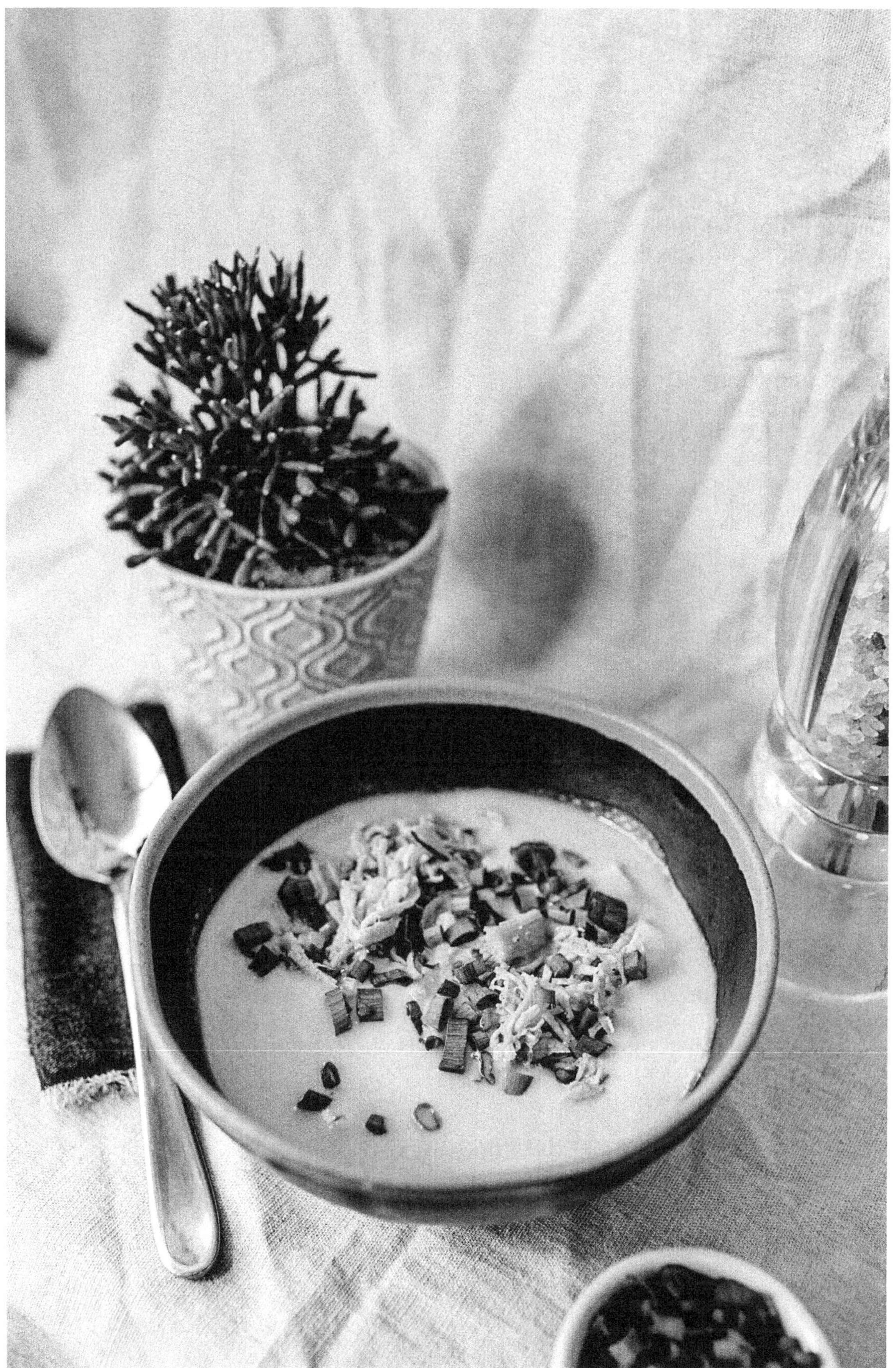

Super Delicious Detox Salad

Yield: 4 Servings
Total Time: 10 Minutes
Prep Time: 10 Minutes
Cook Time: N/A

Ingredients
For Lime Ginger Dressing
½ teaspoon minced pickled ginger
2 tablespoons of olive oil
1 tablespoon maple syrup
4 tablespoon rice vinegar
2 tablespoons fresh lime juice

For Salad
1 large carrot, shredded
5 spring onions
4 cups shredded purple or green cabbage
½ cup roughly chopped fresh parsley
2 tablespoons raisins
1 avocado, sliced
1 cup chopped coriander/ cilantro
½ cup walnuts, chopped

Directions
Toss together carrots, cabbage, coriander, spring onions, and parsley; top with walnuts, raisins, and sliced avocado and drizzle with the dressing. Let marinate for at least 5 minutes before serving.

Whisk together the dressing ingredients until well blended.

Nutritional Information per Serving:
Calories: 286 Total Fat: 22g; Carbs: 21g; Dietary Fiber: 7.5g; Sugars: 9.4g; Protein: 5.5g; Sodium: 117mg

Leafy Greens Stir-Fry in Lemon Coconut Sauce

Yield: 2 Servings
Total Time: 20 Minutes
Prep Time: 10 Minutes
Cook Time: 10 Minutes

Ingredients:
2 tablespoons extra-virgin olive oil
2 small red onions, finely sliced
2-3 garlic cloves, peeled and chopped
1 tablespoon of minced ginger
2 cups squash, seeded, diced
2 cups chopped spinach
2 cup cabbage
1 red or green chili, finely chopped
1 lemon, juiced, and zest
1 teaspoon of lemongrass paste
1 tablespoon soy sauce
A pinch of salt and pepper
1 cup low-fat coconut milk

Directions
Set over medium heat in a large frying pan, heat olive oil, sauté onions for about 3 minutes or until fragrant.

Stir in garlic, ginger, lemongrass, and chili; cook for about 2 minutes, stirring.

Add squash and cook for a few more minutes, then add coconut milk, and simmer till squash is tender.

Toss in the spinach, cabbage, lemon juice, soy sauce, salt, and pepper; cook for 2 minutes.

Nutritional Information Per Serving:
Calories: 356; Total Fat: 22.4g; Net Carbs: 28g; Dietary Fiber: 6g; Sugars: 15g; Protein: 6g; Sodium: 597mg

Spicy Zesty Green Soup with Brown Rice

Yield: 4 Servings
Total Time: 35 Minutes
Prep Time: 5 Minutes
Cook Time: 30 Minutes

Ingredients
2 cups chopped kale
1 cup spinach
2 cups green beans
1 cup brown rice, rinsed
2 yellow onions, chopped
3 cloves garlic
2 tablespoons olive oil
4 to 5 cups vegetable broth
2 lemons, juiced, and zest
1 green chili
¼ teaspoon sea salt
low-fat Greek yogurt

Directions
Add the two tablespoons of olive oil to a large pan and cook the onions over medium heat for about 8 minutes.

In the meantime, cook the rice in a rice cooker until cooked.

In a large soup pot, add onions and oil, cook until soft, add garlic and cook for another minute.

Then add green beans and 4 cups of veggie broth, cook for about 5 minutes, and add kale, spinach, lemon juice, lemon zest, and chili.

Stir frequently. Add another cup of veggie broth if needed.

Once the greens have wilted, add half the rice stirring to combine. Then transfer to a blender or use a stick blender and blitz till smooth.

Transfer back to the pot, add the remainder of the rice, season with salt and pepper, and then serve hot with a spoon full of low-fat greek yogurt

Nutritional Information per Serving:
Calories: 244; Total Fat: 9.2g; Net Carbs: 31.5g; Dietary Fiber: 5.2g; Sugars: 6.5g; Protein: 11.5g; Sodium: 619mg

Delicious Buckwheat with Mushrooms & Green Onions

Yield: 4 Servings
Total Time: 45 Minutes
Prep Time: 10 Minutes
Cook Time: 35 Minutes

Ingredients

1 cup uncooked buckwheat
2 cups of veggie broth
3 cups mushrooms, chopped
2 red onion, chopped
1 cup chopped spring onions
2 cups of cherry tomatoes
2 tablespoons coconut oil
A pinch of salt and pepper

Directions

Quickly toast the buckwheat in a frying pan with a bit of oil for about 5 minutes.

Combine buckwheat and veggie broth in a large pan and bring to a boil; cook for 25 minutes or until soft.

Melt coconut oil in a pan and fry in red onion until tender; stir in mushrooms and cook for about 5 minutes or until golden brown.

Stir in cooked buckwheat and cook for a few more minutes, then remove from heat. Serve topped with freshly chopped cherry tomatoes and spring onions.

Nutrition Infomation per Serving:
Calories: 200; Total Fat: 4.8g; Net Carbs: 35g; Dietary Fiber: 6.1g; Sugars: 4.1g; Protein: 6.75g; Sodium: 470mg

Detox Salad with Lemony Poppy Seed Dressing

Yield: 4 Servings
Total Time: 10 Minutes
Prep Time: 10 Minutes

Ingredients
For Lemony Poppy Seed Dressing
⅓ cup fresh lemon juice
4 tablespoons olive oil
1 teaspoon ginger, minced
1 tablespoon American mustard
1 tablespoon maple syrup
1 clove garlic, minced
Pinch salt and pepper
1 tablespoon poppy seeds

For the Salad
1 carrot, roughly grated
2 cups red cabbage, roughly chopped
½ cup chopped parsley
½ cucumber roughly chopped
2 cups kale
2 tablespoons toasted sunflower seeds
½ cup almonds, chopped

Directions
In a small bowl, whisk together all the dressing ingredients, except poppy seeds, until smooth; add poppy seeds and set aside.

Mix all the salad ingredients in a large bowl; drizzle with the dressing and toss to coat well.

Nutrition Information per Serving
Calories: 260; Total Fat: 19g; Carbs: 19g; Dietary Fiber; 6.5g; Sugars: 8g; Protein: 6.7g; Sodium: 146.7mg

Superfood Detox Blueberry Salad

Yields: 4 Servings
Total Time: 10 Minutes
Prep Time: 10 Minutes
Cook Time: N/A

Ingredients
1 cup fresh blueberries
1 carrot, grated
3 spring onions, chopped
3 cups baby spinach, chopped
1 cup rocket, chopped
2 cups of kale, chopped
½ cup almonds, sliced
2 dates, pitted and diced
1 orange peeled and sliced
1 lemon, juiced
4 tablespoons extra-virgin olive oil

Directions
Mix all the ingredients, except lemon juice and olive oil, in a large bowl.

Whisk together olive oil and lemon juice and then pour over the salad; toss to combine well and serve.

Nutritional Information per Serving:
Calories: 212; Total Fat: 15g; Carbs: 15g; Dietary Fiber: 5g; Sugars: 8.5g; Protein: 5.5g; Sodium: 65.7mg

Cherry Cashew Nuts Salad

Yield: 4 Servings
Total Time: 10 Minutes
Prep Time: 10 Minutes
Cook Time: N/A

Ingredients
For the Salad
½ large cucumber, chopped
1 carrot, grated
3 spring onions, chopped
2 cups lettuce, roughly chopped
2 cups baby spinach, chopped
1 cup of rocket, chopped
1 cup sugar snap peas, sliced
1 cup cherries, halved
100 grams low-fat feta, crumbled
½ cup cashew nuts, toasted, chopped

For the Dressing
3 tablespoons sesame oil
2 lemons, juiced
1 tablespoon rice wine vinegar
1 tablespoon of maple syrup
1 teaspoon American mustard
1 clove garlic, minced
Pinch sea salt and black pepper

Directions
Combine all the salad ingredients in a large bowl. Whisk together all the dressing ingredients in a small bowl until well blended.

Drizzle the dressing over the salad and toss until well coated.

Nutritional Information per Serving:
Calories: 292; Total Fat: 20.1g; Carbs: 17.3g; Dietary Fiber: 4g; Sugars: 7.5g
Protein: 10.2g; Sodium: 149mg

Green Bean & Zucchini Sauté with Feta Cheese & Toasted Almonds

Yield: 2 Servings
Total Time: 20 Minutes
Prep Time: 5 Minutes
Cook Time: 15 Minutes

Ingredients
2 tablespoons extra-virgin olive oil
3 cups green beans, sliced
1 small red onion, chopped
2 garlic cloves
2 medium zucchini, thinly sliced
¼ teaspoon of red chili flakes
60g low-fat feta cheese
A pinch of salt and pepper
2 tablespoons lemon juice
½ cup toasted almonds, chopped

Directions
Add olive oil to a pan set over medium heat. Stir in red onions for about 5 minutes or until fragrant; add in garlic, green beans, zucchini, sea salt, pepper, and red chili flakes and sauté, stirring, for about 10 minutes or until the veggies are tender.

Remove the pan from heat and stir in lemon juice. Serve topped with feta cheese and toasted almonds

Nutritional Information per Serving:
Calories: 292; Total Fat: 19.4g; Net Carbs: 20g; Dietary Fiber: 6g; Sugars: 7.9g; Protein: 11.5g; Sodium: 89.5mg

Vegetables Stir-Fry with Tofu & Coconut Milk

Yield: 4 Servings
Total Time: 25 Minutes
Prep Time: 5 Minutes
Cook Time: 20 Minutes

Ingredients
1 cup of green beans
½ leek, finely chopped
1 medium zucchini/courgette chopped
2 cups firm tofu
1 green bell pepper
1 red bell pepper
2 tablespoons coconut oil
1 can (400g) light coconut milk
2 tablespoons of peanut butter
1 tablespoon of ginger. minced
2 teaspoons of garlic, minced
1 tablespoon Thai green curry paste
A pinch of sea salt and pepper

Directions
Dice zucchini, tofu, bell peppers, leek, tomatoes, and beans in bite-size pieces. Heat the oil in a pan and fry tofu for about 3 minutes. Stir in Thai green curry paste, ginger, peanut butter, and garlic; cook for a few more minutes.

Add beans, leek, zucchini, and bell peppers; fry for 3 more minutes.

Stir in coconut milk and simmer for 10 minutes—season with salt and pepper.

Serve with wild rice.

Nutritional Information Per Serving:
Calories: 316; Total Fat: 23g; Net Carbs: 15.7g; Dietary Fiber: 5.2g; Sugars: 6g; Protein: 15.5g; Sodium: 349mg

Zesty Creamed Corn Salad

Yield: 4 Servings
Total Time: 10 Minutes
Prep Time: 10 Minutes
Cook Time: N/A

Ingredients
3 cups corn kernels
1 red onion, diced
1 red bell pepper, chopped
1 cup chopped cilantro/coriander
½ cup chopped parsley

For the dressing
1 cup low-fat Greek yogurt
1 lime, juiced, and zest
1 teaspoon minced garlic
½ teaspoon cumin seeds
¼ teaspoon chili flakes
Pinch salt and pepper

Directions
In a large bowl, mix all the salad ingredients, then set aside.

Whisk the Greek yogurt, garlic, chili, cumin, salt, pepper, and lime juice in a small bowl.

Then pour the dressing over the salad and toss well; chill in the refrigerator until ready to serve.

Nutritional Information per Serving:
Calories: 228; Total Fat: 4.7g; Net Carbs: 31.7g; Dietary Fiber: 4.5 g; Sugars: 9.25g; Protein: 13.7g; Sodium: 424mg

Crunchy Sweet & Sour Salad

Yield: 4 Servings
Total Time: 10 Minutes
Prep Time: 10 Minutes

For salad:
4 cups red cabbage, finely chopped
1 cup rocket leaves
3 cups fresh baby spinach
5 large radish, finely sliced
1 large carrot, grated
½ small beetroot, grated
¼ cup pistachios, chopped
1 cup fresh basil leaves
1 teaspoon lemon zest

For dressing:
6 tablespoons extra virgin olive oil
1 teaspoon of garlic, minced
¼ cup apple cider vinegar
1 tablespoon Worcestershire sauce
3 tablespoon maple syrup
3 tablespoons freshly squeezed lemon juice

Directions
In a large bowl, combine all salad ingredients and set aside.

In a small pan, whisk together dressing ingredients and cook on low heat for about 5 minutes; remove from heat and allow to cool before pouring over the salad. Toss and then serve, topped with a sprinkle of chopped pistachios.

Nutritional Information per Serving:
Calories: 291; Total Fat: 23g; Carbs: 18g; Dietary Fiber: 6g; Sugars: 10.2g; Protein: 4.9g; Sodium: 114mg

Avocado, Fennel & Feta Salad

Yield: 4 Servings
Total Time: 10 Minutes
Prep Time: 10 Minutes
Cook Time: N/A

Ingredients

1 large avocado, diced
1 red small onion, thinly sliced
1 large fennel bulb, chopped thinly
½ cucumber, chopped
4 medium tomatoes, chopped
1 tablespoon avocado oil
3 tablespoons extra virgin olive oil
2 tablespoons fresh lime juice
½ cup chopped fresh cilantro/coriander
¼ teaspoon chili flakes
½ cup low-fat feta cheese
¼ teaspoon smoked paprika
Pinch of salt and pepper

Directions

Toss together avocado, coriander, red onion, fennel, cucumber, tomatoes, and feta cheese in a large bowl.

In a small bowl, whisk together avocado oil, extra virgin olive oil, lime juice, chili flakes, paprika, and salt; pour over the salad mixture and toss to combine well.

Nutritional Information Per Serving:

Calories: 254; Total Fat: 21.7g; Net Carbs: 11g; Dietary Fiber: 5g; Sugars: 4.7g; Protein: 5.4g; Sodium: 58.7mg

Cleansing Kale Salad

Yield: 4 Servings
Total Time: 10 Minutes
Prep Time: 10 Minutes
Cook Time: N/A

Ingredients
For the dressing:
2 teaspoons whole-grain mustard
1 teaspoon ginger, minced
1 teaspoon garlic, minced
3 tablespoons fresh lemon juice
2 tablespoons apple cider vinegar
⅓ cup olive oil
¼ teaspoon liquid stevia
Pinch of salt and pepper

For the salad:
2 cups broccoli florets
2 cups red cabbage, thinly sliced
2 cups chopped kale
1 cup grated carrot
½ cup fresh basil
1 red bell pepper, sliced into strips
1 avocado, diced
¼ cup chopped parsley
½ cup chopped walnuts
2 tablespoons hemp seeds

Directions
Blend all the dressing ingredients well in a blender, then set aside.

Mix together in a large salad bowl, cabbage, broccoli, carrots, kale, and the sliced bell pepper.

Pour the dressing over the salad; toss well till coated. Add diced avocado, chopped parsley, hemp seeds, and walnuts; toss again until well coated and serve.

Nutritional Information per Serving:
Calories: 393; Total Fat: 34g; Carbs: 18g; Dietary Fiber: 8g; Sugars: 5.2g; Protein: 8.1g; Sodium: 137mg

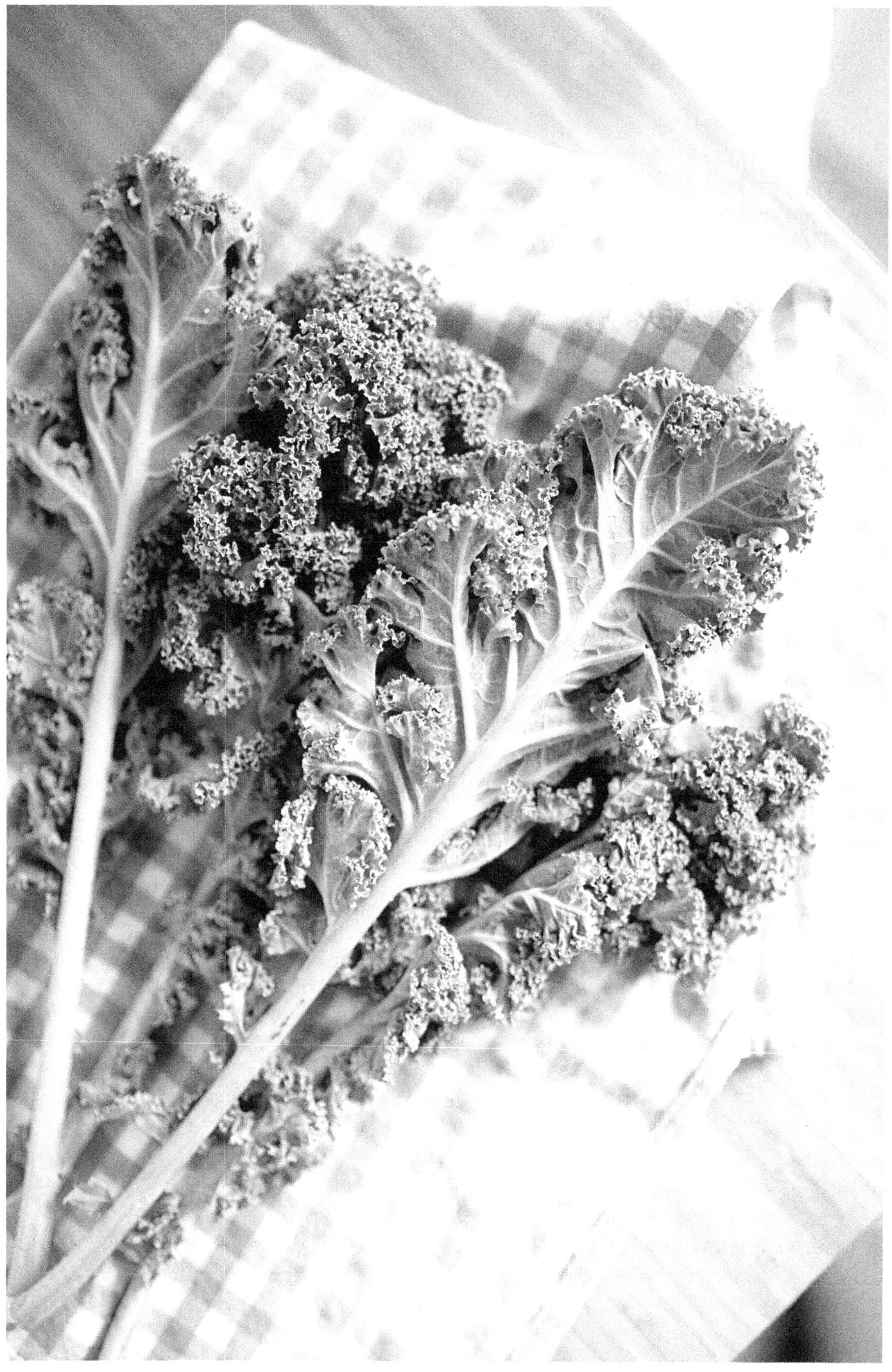

Chickpea Salad Wrap

Yield: 3 Servings
Total Time: 5 Minutes
Prep Time: 5 Minutes
Cook Time: N/A

Ingredients:
1 ½ cups cooked chickpeas
¼ cup toasted sunflower seeds
1 avocado mashed
½ red onion, chopped
1 cup fresh rocket leaves
¼ cup of chopped basil
1 cup baby spinach

Dressing:
2 tablespoons fresh lemon juice
3 tablespoons olive oil
½ tsp regular mustard
1 garlic clove, minced
Pinch salt and black pepper
3 Whole-wheat tortillas

Directions:
In small bowl whisk lemon juice, olive oil, garlic and mustard. In a medium bowl, mash the chickpeas and avocado until smooth.Then in a large bowl, mix all the salad ingredients; toss the dressing in the salad and mix well.

Stuff the mixture into a wrap spread half of the chickpea mixture down the center of each tortilla. Top with the salad, then wrap up like a burrito.

Nutritional Information per Serving:
Calories: 392; Total Fat: 28g; Carbs: 52.2g; Dietary Fiber: 12.6g; Sugars: 5.8g; Protein: 14.6g; Sodium: 347mg

Lemony Squash Salad

Yield: 2 Servings
Total Time: 10 Minutes
Prep Time: 10 Minutes
Cook Time: N/A

Ingredients
½ small red onion, thinly sliced
2 cups baby spinach
2 tbsp chopped chives
2 medium yellow squash, thinly sliced
1 tablespoon balsamic vinegar
3 tablespoons fresh lemon juice
1 tablespoon lemon zest
3 tablespoons olive oil
Pinch salt and black pepper
1 teaspoon hemp seeds
1 teaspoon sesame seeds
½ cup chopped cilantro/coriander

Directions
Mix together red onion, spinach, chives, and squash in a large bowl.

In a small bowl, whisk together vinegar, lemon juice, lemon zest, sea salt, pepper, hemp seeds and sesame seeds until well combined; pour over the squash salad and toss to coat well.

Serve garnished with cilantro/coriander.

Nutritional Information per Serving:
Calories: 242 ;Total Fat: 22g; Carbs: 17.3g; Dietary Fiber: 7.4g; Sugars: 9g; Protein: 7.6g; Sodium: 259mg

Tasty Bean Soup with Tortilla Chips

Yield: 5 Servings
Total Time: 45 Minutes
Prep Time: 10 Minutes
Cook Time: 35 Minutes

Ingredients
2 cups veggie stock
2 large yellow onions, diced
1 tin (400g) tomatoes, chopped
1 tin (400g) of pinto beans, drained
1 tin (400g) kidney beans, drained
2 carrots chopped
1 cup sweetcorn
2 stalks celery, chopped
½ teaspoon chile flakes
3 teaspoons cumin
1 tablespoon minced garlic
½ teaspoon sea salt
1 teaspoon fresh thyme
1 fresh lime, juiced
baked tortilla chips
150g low-fat feta cheese

Directions
Heat oil in a large soup pan, add onions, celery, carrot, and corn. Cook on medium heat for about 5 minutes; add garlic and stir for another minute.

Now add 4 cups of veggie stock to the pan.

Stir in beans, chili flakes, cumin, salt, and tin tomatoes; Bring to a boil, then reduce to a simmer for 25 minutes. Remove from heat and blend using a stick blender until smooth.

Adjust seasoning, add your thyme and simmer on low heat for another 5 minutes

Spoon into serving bowls and drizzle with lime juice and crumbled feta cheese, serve with baked tortilla chips.

Nutritional Information per Serving:
Calories: 279; Total Fat: 8.4g; Carbs: 43g; Dietary Fiber: 9.8g; Sugars: 7.6g; Protein: 16.6g; Sodium: 807mg

Delicious Kale Salad with Grapefruit & Avocado

Yield: 4 Servings
Total Time: 10 Minutes
Prep Time: 10 Minutes
Cook Time: N/A

Ingredients
2 tablespoons fresh grapefruit juice
2 tablespoons fresh orange juice
1 clove garlic, minced
A pinch of sea salt and pepper
½ cup extra virgin olive oil
4 cups shredded kale leaves
1 avocado, sliced
1 grapefruit, sectioned
¼ cup toasted sunflower seeds
½ cup toasted almonds

Directions
Dressing: Whisk together grapefruit juice, orange juice, garlic, salt, and pepper in a small bowl: Let rest for approximately 5 minutes. Then gradually stir in the extra virgin olive oil: set aside.

Add kale to another bowl, drizzle with a splash of the dressing, then massage for about 3 minutes and let sit until tender.

Divide kale among serving plates and top each serving with avocado and grapefruit; sprinkle with toasted almonds and sunflower seeds and drizzle generously with the dressing.

Nutritional Information per Serving:
Calories: 338; Total Fat: 32g; Net Carbs: 15.2g; Dietary Fiber: 6.9g; Sugars: 5.2g; Protein: 7.5g; Sodium: 90.2mg

Edamame & Avocado Salad

Yield: 3 Servings
Total Time: 10 Minutes
Prep Time: 10 Minutes
Cook Time: N/A

Ingredients
3 cups chopped kale
1 cup snow peas, chopped
1 red pepper, chopped
1 yellow pepper, chopped
1 carrot, grated
1 beetroot, grated
1 cup edamame
½ red onion, finely sliced
½ cup of basil, chopped
½ cup of cilantro/coriander, chopped
1 avocado, cubed
Pinch salt

For the vinaigrette:
¼ cup extra-virgin olive oil
1 tablespoon grated fresh ginger
1 lime, juiced, and zest
3 cloves garlic minced
2 tablespoons apple cider vinegar

Directions
Place the kale in a large bowl and sprinkle with the sea salt. Gently massage the kale using your hands until soft and fragrant.

Toss in the remaining salad ingredients until well combined.

Whisk the vinaigrette ingredients, then drizzle over the salad and toss well to combine.

Nutritional Information per Serving:
Calories: 401; Total Fat: 28g; Net Carbs: 33.3g; Dietary Fiber: 14.2g; Sugars: 9.6g; Protein: 12.5g; Sodium: 105mg

Coconut-Black Bean Soup

Yield: 4 Servings
Total Time: 35 Minutes
Prep Time: 5 Minutes
Cook Time: 30 Minutes

Ingredients
1 can (400g) black beans, drained, rinsed
1 can (400g) diced tomatoes
1 can (400g) light coconut milk
1 cup vegetable broth
1 large onion
3 cloves garlic, minced
1 tablespoon ground turmeric
1 tablespoon ground cumin
2 teaspoons ginger, minced
½ teaspoon of chili flakes
2 cloves
1 pinch salt and pepper
4 tablespoons of chopped cilantro/coriander

Directions
In a saucepan, combine together all the ingredients and bring to a gentle boil.
Lower heat and simmer, covered, for about 30 minutes.
Remove from heat and serve in a bowl with a sprinkle of fresh coriander.

Nutrition Information per Serving:
Calories: 256; Total Fat: 7.75g; Net Carbs: 28.6g; Dietary Fiber: 11.5g; Sugar: 6g; Protein: 9.7g; Sodium: 413mg

Millet Stir Fry with Veggies

Yield: 3 Servings
Total Time: 30 Minutes
Prep Time: 10 Minutes
Cook Time: 20 Minutes

Ingredients
1 cup millet
1 small red onion, chopped
1 green chili, chopped
1 tablespoon ginger, minced
2 cloves garlic, minced
1 cup chopped red and yellow bell peppers
1 zucchini, chopped
1 carrot, chopped
1 teaspoon coriander powder
1 teaspoon cumin powder
1 teaspoon turmeric powder
Pinch of salt and pepper
1 tablespoon olive oil
fresh coriander/cilantro leaves
fresh chives, chopped

Directions
Wash millet under running water and soak for at least 8 minutes.

Rinse the millet and drain; add to the pan along with two cups of water. Cover and cook for about 10 minutes or until liquid is absorbed and millet is tender.

Meanwhile, heat oil in a pot and cook in garlic, ginger, and green chili for 1 minute; stir in onions and spices and cook for 2 minutes. Then add veggies and cook for about 7 mins. Stir in the millet, and season with salt and pepper.

Fluff and serve topped with fresh chives and fresh coriander.

Nutritional Information per Serving:
Calories: 180; Total Fat: 5.6g; Net Carbs: 26.8g; Dietary Fiber: 4.7g; Sugars: 3.6g
Protein: 4.7g; Sodium: 78.6mg

Shaved Veggie Salad with Hemp Seeds

Yield: 2 Servings
Total Time: 5 Minutes
Prep Time: 5 Minutes
Cook Time: N/A

Ingredients
4 cups spinach
2 radishes, sliced thinly
1 small yellow squash, sliced thinly
1 red beetroot, thinly sliced
1 cucumber, thinly sliced/ ribboned
1 small carrot, thinly sliced/ ribboned
2 tablespoon hemp seeds
2 tablespoon extra-virgin olive oil
1 lemon, juiced
1 teaspoon of American mustard
Pinch salt and pepper

Directions:
In a small bowl, whisk lemon juice, mustard, and olive oil.

Then, mix the spinach and veggies in a large bowl, pour over the dressing, toss to combine, season with salt and pepper, and top with hemp seeds.

Nutritional Information per Serving:
Calories: 243; Total Fat: 20g; Carbs: 15g; Dietary Fiber: 6g; Sugars: 9g; Protein: 7g; Sodium: 215mg

Healthy Millet Lettuce Wraps

Yield: 2 Servings
Total Time: 30 Minutes
Prep Time: 10 Minutes
Cook Time: 20 Minutes

Ingredients

4 leaves lettuce
½ cup millet
1 teaspoon coconut oil
¾ cup water
1 small red onion, chopped
2 cloves garlic, minced
1 teaspoon ginger, minced
1 teaspoon paprika
2 tablespoons fresh lime juice
1 tablespoon chopped cilantro/coriander
Pinch salt and pepper
1 carrot, grated

Directions

In a pan, toast millet for about 3 minutes or until fragrant; transfer to a plate and set aside. Add coconut oil to the pan and sauté in red onion, ginger, and garlic for about 3 minutes or until fragrant. Stir in toasted millet, lime juice, sea salt, paprika, and water; simmer for about 10 minutes or until the liquid is absorbed. Remove from heat.

Divide carrots among the lettuce leaves, top each with the millet mixture with fresh coriander, dash more lime juice, and roll to form wraps and serve.

Nutrition info Per Serving:

Calories: 105; Total Fat: 2.5g; Net Carbs: 18.5g; Dietary Fiber: 3.5g; Sugars: 2.2g; Protein: 3g; Sodium: 112mg

Vegan Red Lentil Soup

Yield: 5 Servings
Total Time: 45 Minutes
Prep Time: 10 Minutes
Cook Time: 35 Minutes

Ingredients
5 cups low-sodium vegetable broth
2 tablespoons minced garlic
1 ½ cups chopped red onion
1 teaspoon paprika
1 teaspoon ground coriander
1 teaspoon cumin seeds
½ teaspoon pepper
1 ½ cups red lentils
2 carrots, chopped
1 leek, chopped
Fresh lemon juice
Fresh basil leaves

Directions
Add vegetable stock to a saucepan and stir in garlic, onion, paprika, pepper, and ground coriander; bring to a gentle boil. Add leek, carrots, and cook for 10 minutes; then add lentils.

Cook, covered, for 35 minutes or until lentils are tender. Remove from heat and blend with a stick blender until smooth. Return to heat and simmer for a few more minutes.

Serve in bowls garnished with fresh lemon and fresh basil leaves.

Nutrition Information per Serving
Calories: 243; Total Fat: 3.6g; Carbs: 40.5g; Dietary Fiber: 7.2g;Sugars: 2.6g; Protein: 15.2g; Sodium: 689mg

Spicey Baked Sweet Potato and Spring Onion Salad

Yield: 4 Servings
Total Time: 40 Minutes
Prep Time: 10 Minutes
Cook Time: 30 Minutes

Ingredients
4 sweet potatoes, peeled, diced
4 sliced spring onions
1 medium red bell pepper, chopped
1 medium yellow bell pepper, chopped
2 tablespoons basil leaves
1 green chili, chopped
1 teaspoon grated orange zest
2 teaspoons ground cumin
¼ cup apple cider vinegar
4 tablespoons extra-virgin olive oil
¼ teaspoon sea salt and black pepper

Directions
Preheat your oven to 350ºF/177ºC

Place sweet potatoes on a baking sheet and drizzle with half of the oil; sprinkle with salt and pepper and toss to coat well. Bake in the preheated oven for about 20 minutes, toss in the red and yellow bell peppers and bake for another 10 minutes or until tender.

Meanwhile, add the remaining oil to the blender along with the chili, vinegar, orange zest, cumin, salt, pepper, and blend until smooth.

Remove the potatoes and bell peppers from the oven and sprinkle with basil and spring onions. Drizzle with the dressing and toss to coat well.

Nutrition info Per Serving:
Calories: 376; Total Fat: 20.6g; Net Carbs: 46.5g; Dietary Fiber: 9.7g; Sugars: 17g; Protein: 5.74g; Sodium: 139mg

Mains

AND SIDES

"You carry the key to your own happiness. Unlock your inner potential"

Monty's Dream's

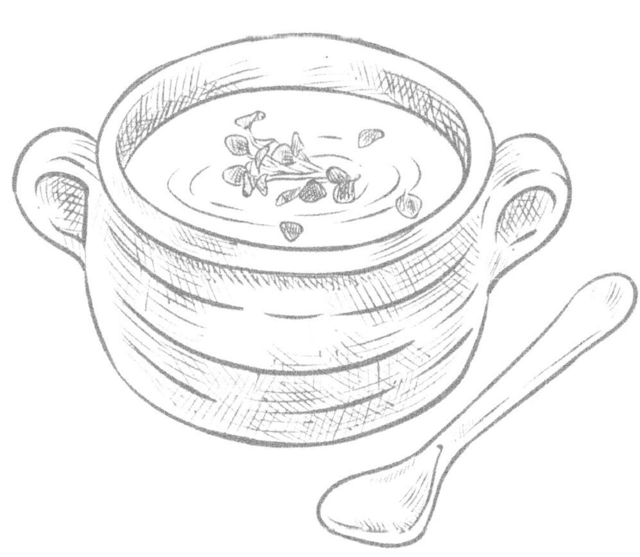

Coconut-Crumbed Chicken Bake with a Kick

Yield: 4 Servings
Total Time: 45 Minutes
Prep Time: 15 Minutes
Cook Time: 35 Minutes

Ingredients
4 skinless chicken breasts
1 butternut squash, diced
4 tablespoons gluten-free breadcrumb
3 tablespoons desiccated coconut
2 eggs
2 tablespoons extra-virgin olive oil
½ teaspoon of chili flakes
¼ teaspoon sea salt and black pepper
1 teaspoon of fresh thyme
2 large red bell peppers, chopped
lime wedges
handful coriander, chopped

Directions
Preheat oven to 400ºF/205ºC
Toss the butternut squash in a large bowl with olive oil; spread out in a roasting pan, sprinkle with salt, and roast for about 30 minutes, turning once.

Crack the eggs into a bowl.

Then, mix bread crumbs, coconut, chili flakes, sea salt, and pepper in another bowl.

Dip the chicken into the bowl of eggs and then into the bowl of shredded coconut, pressing into the crumb mixture.

Place the chicken on another baking tray and bake for 20 minutes, turning halfway.

Toss the red bell peppers into the roasted butternut squash, then sprinkle with thyme, bake for another 3 minutes.

Check the chicken is cooked through then serve garnished with lime wedges and coriander.

Nutritional Info per Serving:
Calories: 405; Total Fat: 24.2g; Carbs: 31.2g; Dietary Fiber: 8.5g; Sugars: 9.2g; Protein: 41.9g; Sodium: 173mg

Grilled Chickpeas Wraps with Salsa Crema

Yield: 4 Servings
Total Time: 20 Minutes
Prep Time: 10 Minutes
Cook Time: 10 Minutes

Ingredients

For Salsa Crema:

1 lemon juiced and zest
½ cup raw walnuts
½ cup raw cashews
½ cup your favorite roasted salsa
½ cup silk cashew milk

For Burritos:

4 whole-wheat wraps
¾ cup cooked chickpeas
¾ cup cooked brown rice
1 avocado, mashed
½ cup low-fat cheese of your choice
Sea salt
Chopped cilantro/coriander

Directions

Blend all cream ingredients in a blender until smooth, then set aside.

In a large bowl, combine cooked rice, chickpeas, and salt, then divide the mixture between four tortillas and top with mashed avocado and low-fat cheese.

Fold to enclose and wrap the filling, placing seam side down on a frying pan.

Cook on medium to low heat for approximately 5 minutes or until the tortillas are browned; flip over, and cook the other side till browned. Place the tortillas on serving plates and drizzle each with salsa crema. Serve garnished with chopped cilantro/coriander.

Nutrition Information per Serving

Calories: 486; Total Fat: 25g; Carbs: 52g; Dietary Fiber: 8.7g; Sugars: 4g; Protein: 15.7g; Sodium: 596mg

Raw Zucchini Pasta with Tasty Avocado Sauce

Yield: 2 Servings
Total Time: 25 Minutes
Prep Time: 25 Minutes
Cook Time: N/A

Ingredients
2 large zucchini, spiralized
2 avocados
1 garlic clove
2 tablespoons fresh lemon juice
½ teaspoon salt
¼ teaspoon ground pepper
½ cup fresh basil leaves
¼ cup fresh coriander/cilantro

Directions
Add the spiralized zucchini to a large bowl and sprinkle with salt; set aside for at least 20 minutes.

In a blender, blend the remaining ingredients until smooth and creamy.

Drain the zucchini and stir in avocado cream; mix to coat well and serve.

Top with a few more fresh basil leaves

Nutrition Information per Serving
Calories: 270; Total Fat: 22.4g; Carbs: 20.2g; Dietary Fiber: 12.1g; Sugars: 4g; Protein: 5g; Sodium: 169mg

Pan-Seared Salmon with Crunchy Cabbage Slaw & Toasted Almonds

Yield: 4 Servings
Total Time: 20 Minutes
Prep Time: 10 Minutes
Cook Time: 10 Minutes

Ingredients

4 Salmon skin-on
1 ½ tablespoons olive oil
4 cups thinly sliced red cabbage
1 carrot, grated
1 teaspoon maple syrup
1 lime, juiced, and zest
4 spring onions, chopped
1 red bell pepper, thinly sliced
1 yellow bell pepper, thinly sliced
½ cup fresh mint leaves
½ cup fresh coriander leaves
½ cup chopped toasted almonds
Lime wedges

Directions

Heat half tablespoon of oil in a frying pan over medium heat; place in salmon, skin side down, and cook for about 5 minutes or until the skin is crisp; turn over to cook the other side for about 3 minutes or until cooked through.

In the meantime, whisk together maple syrup, lime juice, lime zest, salt, and the remaining oil until well blended; add in cabbage, spring onions, bell peppers, carrot, mint, and coriander. Stir in salt and pepper.

Divide the cabbage slaw among serving plates and top each serving with salmon. Sprinkle with chopped toasted almonds and garnish with lime wedges.

Nutritional Information per Serving:

Calories: 365; Total Fat: 17g; Carbs: 14.7g; Dietary Fiber: 4.5g; Sugars: 6g; Protein: 39g; Sodium: 205mg

Zesty Ginger Carrot Noodles

Yield: 4 Servings
Total Time: 20 Minutes
Prep Time: 5 Minutes
Chill Time: 20 Minutes

Ingredients
4 large carrots, spiralized
1 teaspoon garlic, minced
1 tablespoon ginger, minced
½ teaspoon paprika
2 tablespoons fresh coriander/cilantro
3 tablespoons walnut oil
2 tablespoons fresh lime juice
Pinch salt and pepper

Directions
Wash, then spiralize the carrots to make thin noodles.

Add ginger to a large bowl, then add paprika, coriander/cilantro, garlic, and fresh lime juice. Stir in the walnut oil until well combined, season with salt and pepper. Pour the dressing over the carrot noodles and toss to coat well. Refrigerate for at least 20 minutes; This allows the flavors to mature before serving.

Nutritional Information per Serving:
Calories: 120; Total Fat: 9g; Carbs: 6.2g; Dietary Fiber: 1.9g; Sugars: 3.5g; Protein: 0.9g; Sodium: 87mg

Delicious Slow Cooker Quinoa-Lentil Tacos

Yield: 6 Servings
Total Time: 6 Hours 10 Minutes
Prep Time: 10 Minutes
Cook Time: 6 Hours

Ingredients
1 cup lentils, soaked and rinsed
¼ cup quinoa, rinsed
2 cloves garlic, minced
200g (7oz) chopped tomatoes
3 cups veggie stock
1 tablespoon Cajun spice
1 teaspoon fresh thyme
4 spring onions/scallions
Salt and pepper
6 corn taco shells
1 avocado

Directions
In a slow cooker, combine all ingredients, except taco shells, salt, and pepper; cook on a high for about 30 minutes, stirring occasionally.

Then set on low for about 5 hours. Make sure to check now and then and stir.

Season with salt and pepper and serve in taco shells with tomatoes, lettuce, spring onions, and avocado.

Nutrition Information per Serving
Calories: 258; Total Fat: 6.1g; Carbs: 34.1g; Dietary Fiber; 5.8g; Sugars: 1.8g; Protein: 10.1g; Sodium: 533mg

Chicken Cacciatore with Brown Rice

Yield: 4 Servings
Total Time: 60 Minutes
Prep Time: 15 Minutes
Cook Time: 45 Minutes

Ingredients
4 (150g/ 5oz) chicken thighs, skinless
2 cups mushrooms, sliced
2 tablespoons olive oil
1 cup olives, pitted
200g (7oz) cherry tomatoes
1 tablespoon of tomato paste
1 cup chicken stock
½ cup white wine vinegar
1 carrot, peeled, chopped
1 yellow bell pepper, chopped
1 large onion, thinly sliced
1 red bell pepper, chopped
4 garlic cloves, chopped
4 large ripe tomatoes, chopped
2 tablespoons chopped fresh oregano
2 tablespoons grated Parmesan cheese
2 tablespoons chopped fresh basil
2 cups cooked brown rice

Directions
Sprinkle chicken with salt and pepper; heat oil in a large frying pan over medium-high heat and then cook in chicken for about 4 minutes per side. Transfer to a dish and keep warm.
Add the mushrooms, onions, bell peppers to the pan and cook for a few minutes or until tender; transfer to a large bowl.

Add the remaining oil to the pan; Stir in garlic and chopped tomatoes for about 4 minutes or until tender. Stir in carrots and herbs for about 2 minutes, and then add in wine vinegar and tomato paste. Cook for about 5 minutes or until liquid is reduced by half.

Return the chicken, mushrooms, and veggies to the pan and stir in olives and cherry tomatoes. Then add the chicken stock; bring the mixture to a gentle boil. Then lower heat and simmer.

Make sure to cover with a lid for about 30 minutes or until the chicken is cooked. Stir in chopped oregano.

Serve hot with cooked brown rice, garnish with chopped basil and parmesan cheese!

Nutritional Information per Serving:
Calories: 531; Total Fat: 14.2g; Net Carbs: 46.4g; Dietary Fiber: 7.4g; Sugars: 12.7g; Protein: 54.3g;Sodium: 326mg

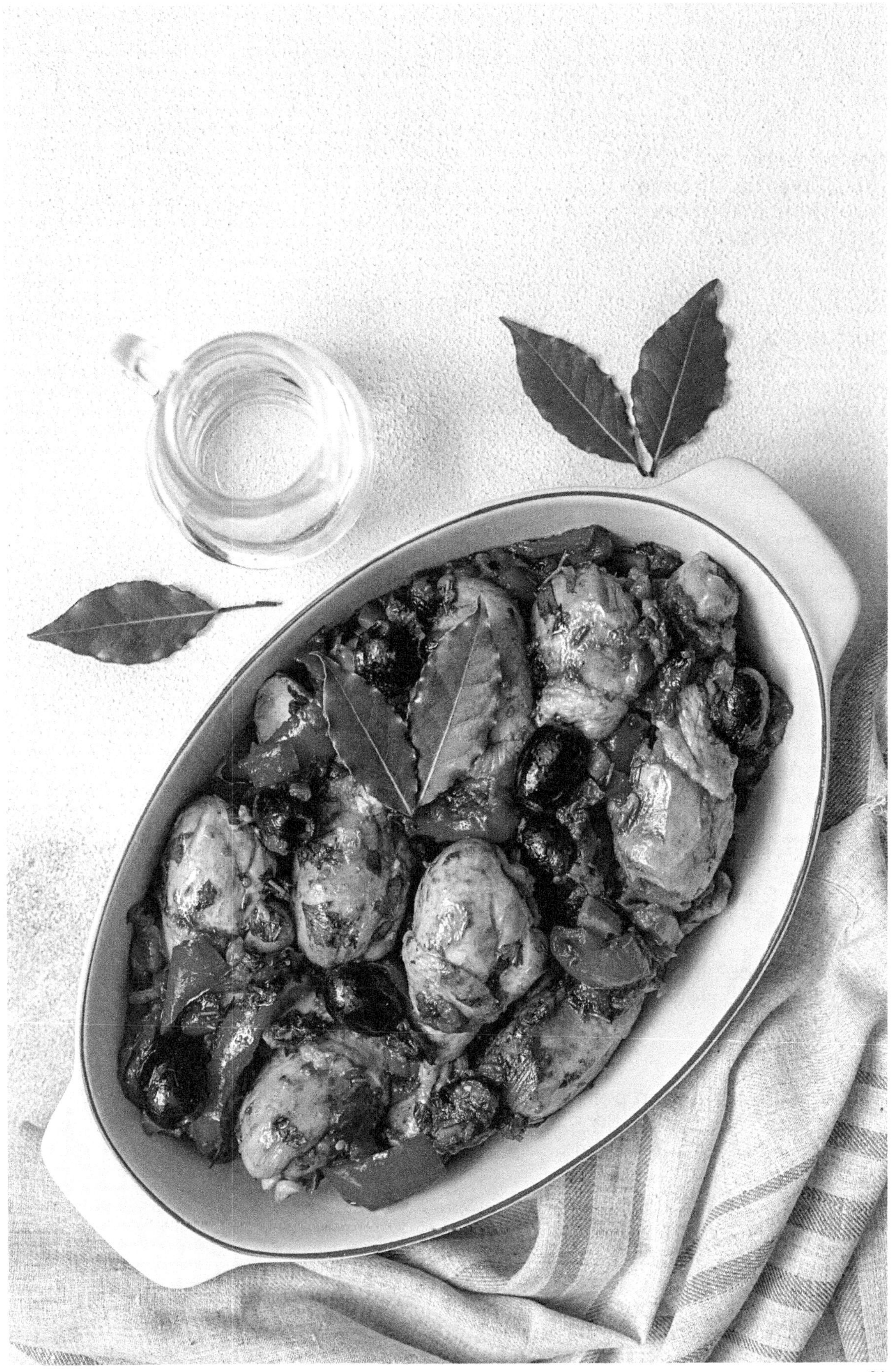

Indian Spiced Lentils

Yield: 4 Servings
Total Time: 50 Minutes
Prep Time: 5 Minutes
Cook Time: 45 Minutes

Ingredients
3 cups veggie stock
1 cup frozen corn and peas
1 cup red lentils
3 tablespoons minced garlic
1 teaspoon turmeric
2 teaspoon cumin
2 cloves
1 teaspoon curry powder
1 cinnamon stick
½ teaspoon salt and pepper
1 bay leaf
1 cup basmati rice
1 ⅕ cups water

Directions
Rinse and drain both lentils and rice.

Heat oil in a large pot over medium-high heat, and add all the spices and garlic; sauté for about 2 minutes. Then add 3 cups of veggie stock, bring it to a boil, add the lentils. Cook for roughly 35 minutes or until lentils start to go tender. Add frozen corn and peas to lentils and cook for another 10 minutes.

Meanwhile, cook the rice in a rice cooker with a pinch of salt and a bay leaf. Serve the lentil-veggie stew over the rice. Garnish with fresh coriander.

Nutritional Information per Serving:
Calories: 355 Total Fat: 1.6g; Carbs: 71g; Dietary Fiber: 26g; Sugars: 3.2g; Protein: 16.4g; Sodium: 281mg

Tasty Mushroom Marinara with Pasta

Yield: 4 Servings
Total Time: 45 Minutes
Prep Time: 5 Minutes
Cook Time: 40 Minutes

Ingredients:
½ cup of red wine
1 onion, chopped
3-4 cups sliced mushrooms
4 garlic cloves, minced
½ teaspoon cayenne pepper
1 ½ teaspoon dried thyme
1 ½ teaspoon dried oregano
1 teaspoon dried basil
1 tin chopped tomatoes
2 cups chopped cherry tomatoes
300g (10oz) whole-wheat pasta
120g (4oz) of low-fat feta

Directions:
Cook onions in a dash of oil for about 2 minutes; stir in mushrooms and garlic and cook for about 5 minutes or until mushrooms are lightly browned, and onion is tender.

Stir in thyme, oregano, cayenne pepper, basil, tin tomatoes, cherry tomatoes, and red wine; simmer for about 35 minutes.

Follow your package instructions to cook the pasta; drain and serve with a sprinkling of low-fat feta cheese or another cheese of your choice.

Nutrition Information per Serving
Calories: 360; Total Fat: 5.5g; Carbs: 54.6g; Dietary Fiber: 2g; Sugars: 4.7g; Protein: 17.1g; Sodium: 18.9mg

Chicken and Buckwheat Salad Served with Chili-Tomato Salsa

Yield: 4 Servings
Total Time: 20 Minutes
Prep Time: 5 Minutes
Cook Time: 15 Minutes

Ingredients:
¼ cup fresh lemon juice
2 teaspoons ground turmeric
2 tablespoons extra-virgin olive oil
4 chicken breasts, skinless, boneless
3 cups chopped baby spinach
1 teaspoon ginger, minced
1 teaspoon garlic, minced
1 large red onion, sliced
1 leek, finely chopped
1 cup buckwheat
Bay leaf
For the salsa
3 large tomatoes, finely chopped
2 tablespoons capers, finely chopped
1 red chili, finely chopped
¼ cup fresh lemon juice
½ cup basil, finely chopped
1 avocado, diced

Directions
Make the salsa: mix avocado, chopped tomato, capers, chili, lemon juice, and basil in a large bowl.
Preheat your oven to 450°F/230°C

In a large bowl, mix lemon juice, 1 teaspoon turmeric, garlic, and a splash of extra virgin olive oil; add the chicken and stir to combine well. Marinate for about 10 minutes.
Set an ovenproof pan over medium heat and add the chicken; cook for about 4 minutes per side or until lightly browned. Transfer to the preheated oven and bake for about 10 minutes.

Remove the chicken from the oven and keep warm.

Fry ginger, leeks, and red onion in a splash of extra virgin olive oil until tender.

Follow package instructions to cook buckwheat with the remaining turmeric and bay leaf.

Serve the buckwheat with chicken, veggies, baby spinach, and salsa.

Nutritional Information per Serving:
Calories: 499; Total Fat: 24.5g; Net Carbs: 23g; Dietary Fiber: 9.4g; Sugars: 5.3g; Protein: 43.2g; Sodium: 327mg

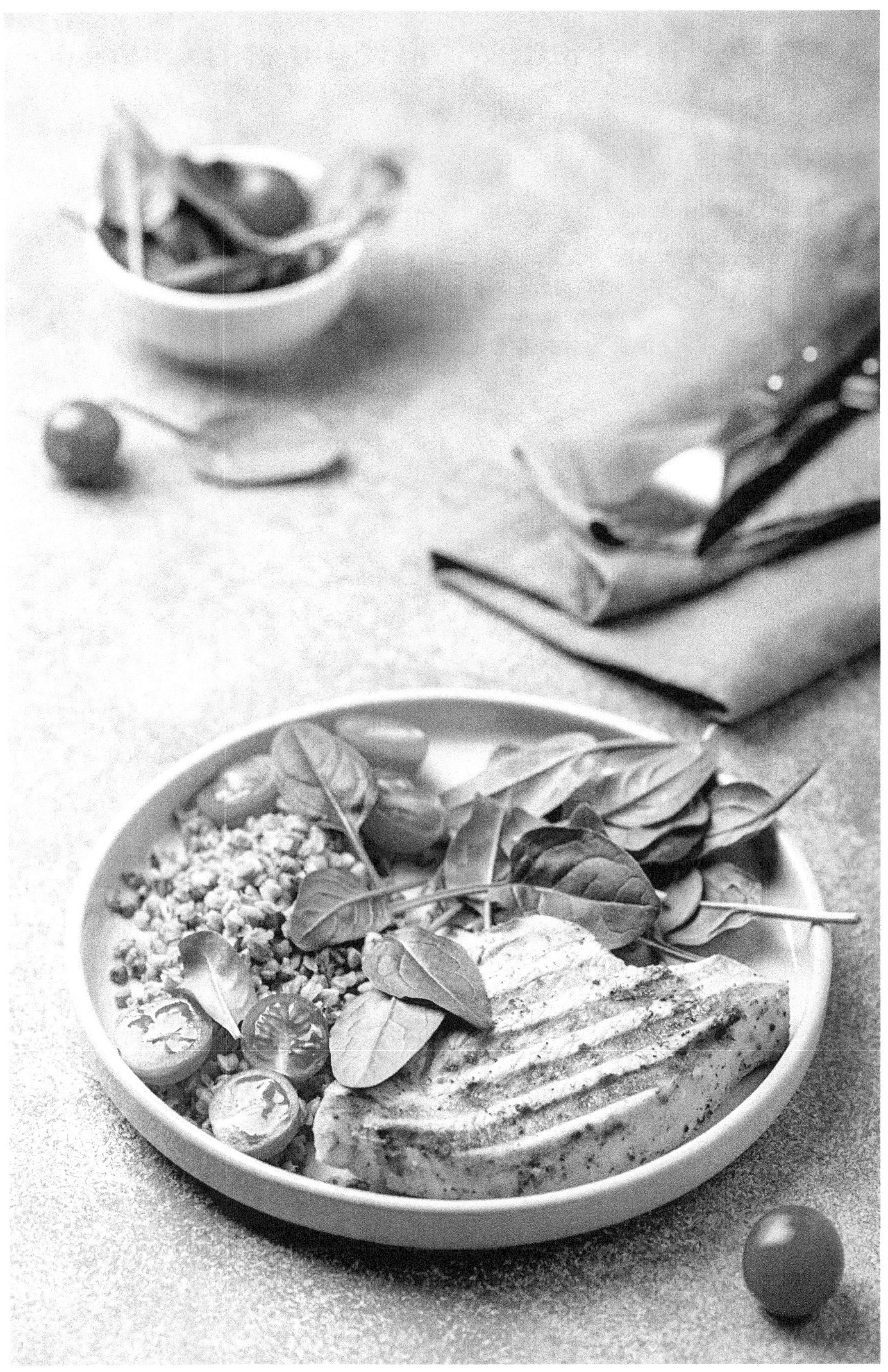

Herby Spaghetti with Garlic and Olives

Yield: 4 Servings
Total Time: 25 Minutes
Prep Time: 10 Minutes
Cook Time: 15 Minutes

Ingredients:
500 grams spaghetti
½ cup extra virgin olive oil
1 teaspoon garlic minced
1 red onion, chopped
2 red chilies, seeds removed
¼ cup fresh parsley, coarsely chopped
½ cup fresh basil, coarsely chopped
1 cup fresh olives, pitted and chopped in half
¼ cup grated parmesan cheese
Pinch salt

Directions:
Boil a pot of salted water and then add the spaghetti; cook until the spaghetti is just soft.

In the meantime, make the sauce. Add garlic, chili, onions oil to a frying pan. Gently cook for about 3 minutes.

Stir in olives, chopped parsley, and basil.

Drain the spaghetti but reserve 1/4 cup cooking water. Stir the spaghetti into the frying pan; stir well, ensuring it's coated completely. Add some of the starchy spaghetti water. Cook for another minute, stirring well.

Serve with grated parmesan cheese, fresh basil, and parsley.

Nutritional Information per Serving:
Calories: 378; Total Fat: 8.6 g; Carbs: 52.9 g; Dietary Fiber: 3.7g; Sugars: 3.2 g; Protein: 12.4 g; Sodium: 985 mg

Baked Potato & Chili Beans

Yield: 4 Servings
Total Time: 1 Hour 20 Minutes
Prep Time: 20 Minutes
Cook Time: 60 Minutes

Ingredients:
4 large potatoes, washed skin on
1 tin (400g/14oz) Pinto beans
1 tin (400g/14oz) tomatoes
Canola oil
1 yellow onion, chopped
1 red pepper, chopped
1 cup fresh coriander, finely chopped
1 tablespoon cumin powder
1 teaspoon smoked paprika
1 teaspoon cinnamon powder
1 fresh red chili, deseeded and finely chopped

Directions
Preheat your oven to 425°F/220°C. Wash the potatoes, then pat dry. Cook the potatoes in the microwave for 5 minutes. Then coat with canola oil and sprinkle with salt and pepper.

Arrange the potatoes on a roasting tray. Sprinkle with a pinch each of cumin, cinnamon, and paprika.

Bake for about 50 minutes to 60 minutes until soft; Flip them over every 25 minutes or so.

Add 1 tablespoon of oil to a pan and sauté the onion, peppers, coriander, chili, and spices.

Stir in the beans together with the tin of tomatoes. Simmer for half an hour. Once the potatoes are baked, cut in half and mash a knob of butter inside. Teasing the inside of the potato with a fork, light and fluffy. Pour the sauce and beans over the potatoes with add fresh coriander to garnish.

Nutritional Information per Serving:
Calories: 288; Total Fat: 2.6g; Carbs: 56.9g; Dietary Fiber: 11.4g; Sugars: 6.2g; Protein: 10.4g; Sodium: 534mg

Green Beans with Ginger & Toasted Almonds

Yield: 2 Servings
Total Time: 15 Minutes
Prep Time: 5 Minutes
Cook Time: 10 Minutes

Ingredients
2 tablespoons extra-virgin olive oil
3 cups green beans, sliced
1 cup chopped red onion
2 garlic cloves, minced
1 teaspoon ginger, minced
A pinch of salt and pepper
2 tablespoons lemon juice
½ cup scallions/spring onions
1 cup sliced toasted almonds

Directions
Add olive oil to a frying pan set over medium heat.

Stir in red onions for about 5 minutes or until fragrant; add in garlic, green beans, ginger, sea salt, pepper, and sauté for about 8 minutes or until the veggies are tender.

Remove the pan from heat and stir in lemon juice and spring onions.

Serve topped with sliced toasted almonds.

Nutritional Information per Serving:
Calories: 239; Total Fat: 20 g; Net Carbs: 17.3 g; Dietary Fiber: 7.4g; Sugars: 7 g; Protein: 7.5 g; Sodium: 185 mg

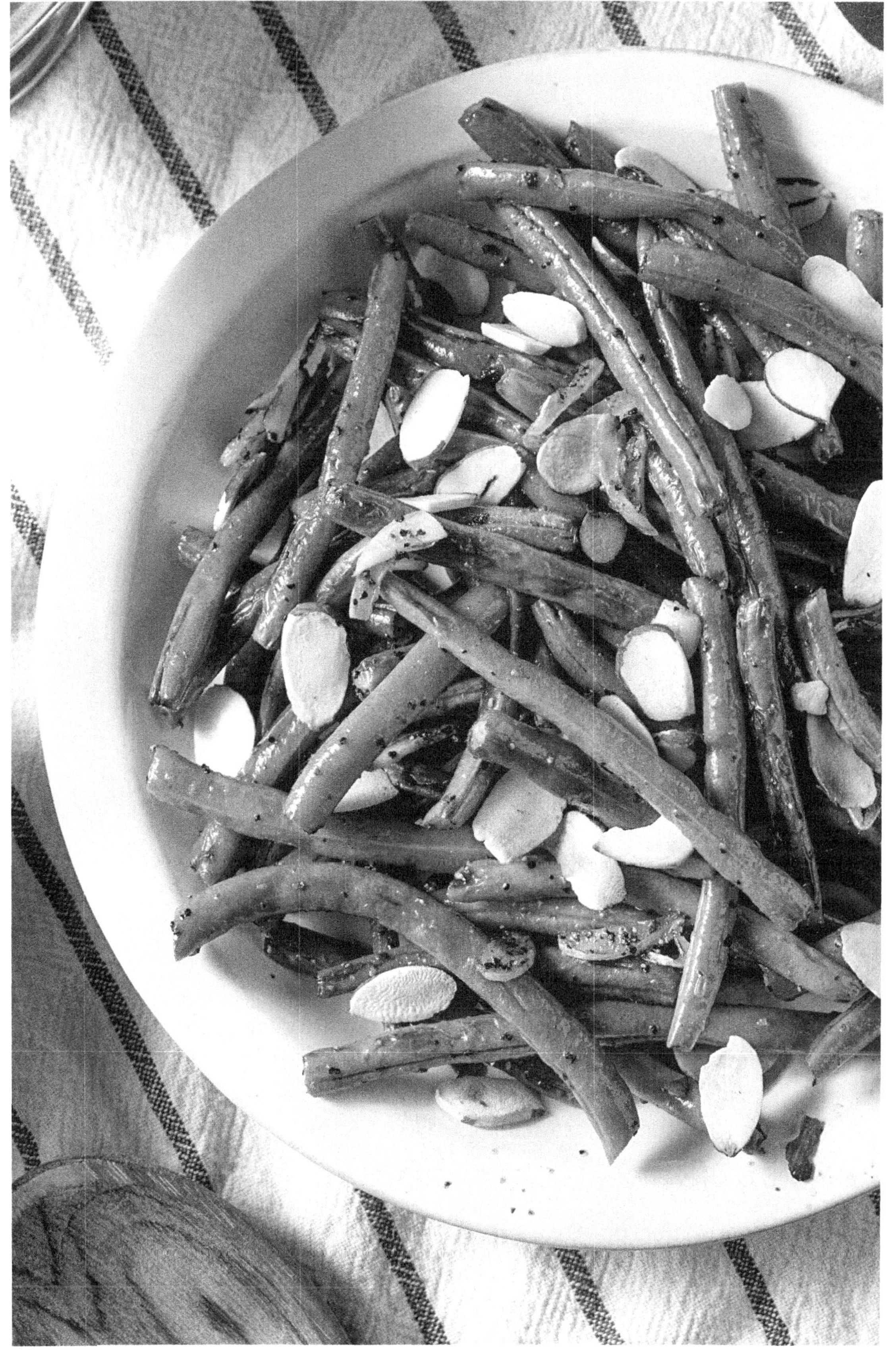

Spiced Veggie Curry with Rice

Yield: 4 Servings
Total Time: 30 Minutes
Prep Time: 15 Minutes
Cook Time: 15 Minutes

Ingredients
2 green zucchini, chopped
1 cup frozen peas
1 cup frozen corn
1 cup green beans, chopped
½ cup chopped coriander
1 small onion
1 cup rice

For the sauce:
1 onion, chopped
1 teaspoon ground turmeric
3 clove garlic, finely chopped
1 red chili, deseeded and chopped
1 teaspoon ginger paste
400ml (1.7 cups) low-fat coconut milk
1 tablespoon curry powder
Juice of 1 lime
zest of lime

Directions
Start by making the sauce

Combine all the sauce ingredients in your food processor and pulse until perfectly smooth.

Fry onions in a pan with a dash of oil for 2 minutes, then stir in the remaining veggies and cook for another 5 minutes. Then add the spicy coconut sauce, simmer on low to medium heat for approximately 15 minutes, or until veggies are cooked.

Cook the rice as per packet instructions.

Garnish with fresh coriander and a slice lime.

Nutritional Information per Serving:
Calories: 334; Total Fat: 12.2g; Carbs: 57.4g; Dietary Fiber: 5.8g; Sugars: 7.6g; Protein: 4.8g; Sodium: 38mg

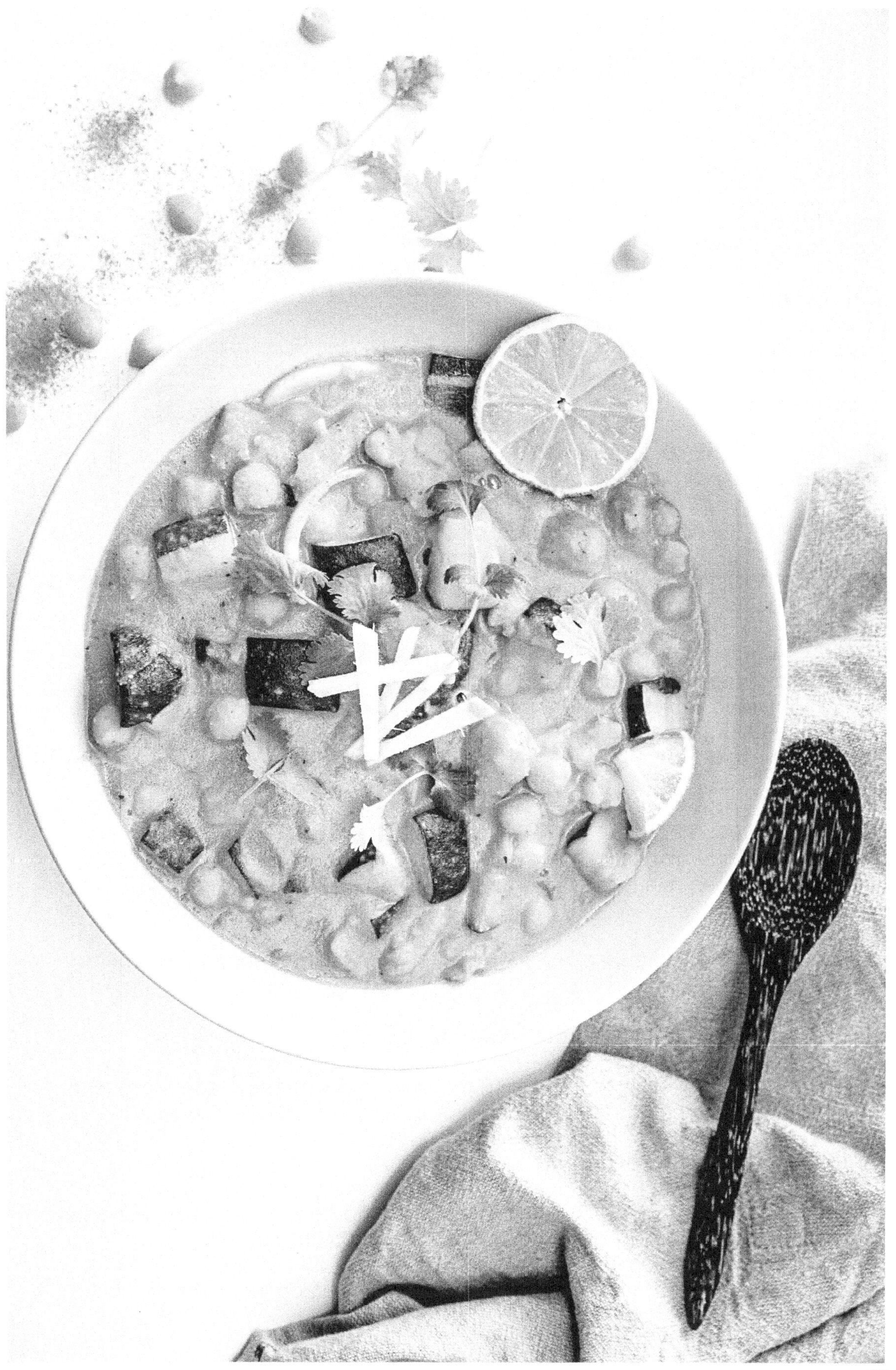

Superfast Moroccan Lamb & Couscous

Yield: 4 Servings
Total Time: 15 Minutes
Prep Time: 5 Minutes
Cook Time: 10 Minutes

Ingredients
CousCous Salad
1 cup chicken stock
1 cup couscous
1 red onion, diced
1 carrot, grated
400g (14oz) tin chickpeas, drained, rinsed
1 cup fresh coriander leaves, roughly chopped
2 cups rocket, roughly chopped
1 cup baby spinach, roughly chopped
1 tsp lime zest
1 tbsp extra virgin olive oil
Lime wedges, to serve

Moroccan lamb
2 tablespoons fresh coriander
400g (14oz) lamb
3 tablespoons Moroccan spices
2 tbsp extra virgin olive oil

Mint yogurt
1 tablespoon lemon juice
1 cup low-fat Greek yogurt
2 tablespoons fresh mint, finely chopped

Directions
In a pan, boil the chicken stock on high heat. Remove from heat, then add the couscous, cover, and set aside.

In the meantime, make the Moroccan spiced lamb.

Heat a tablespoon of olive oil in a frying pan over medium heat; add Moroccan spices and stir. Then add the lamb, cook for a few minutes on each side.

Transfer to a plate and keep warm.

Fluff the couscous with a fork. Chop all the salad ingredients and toss into a large bowl; add the couscous and toss again. Drizzle with a little olive oil.

Make Minted yogurt: Combine low-fat Greek yogurt, lemon juice, and mint in a bowl. Then season with salt and pepper.

Serve the sliced lamb over the couscous, garnish with lime, and a sprinkle of fresh coriander. Add a few cherry tomatoes if you wish.

Nutrition Information per Serving
Calories: 578; Total Fat: 23.4g; Carbs: 48.5g; Dietary Fiber: 8.6g; Sugars: 6g; Protein: 43.7g; Sodium: 287mg

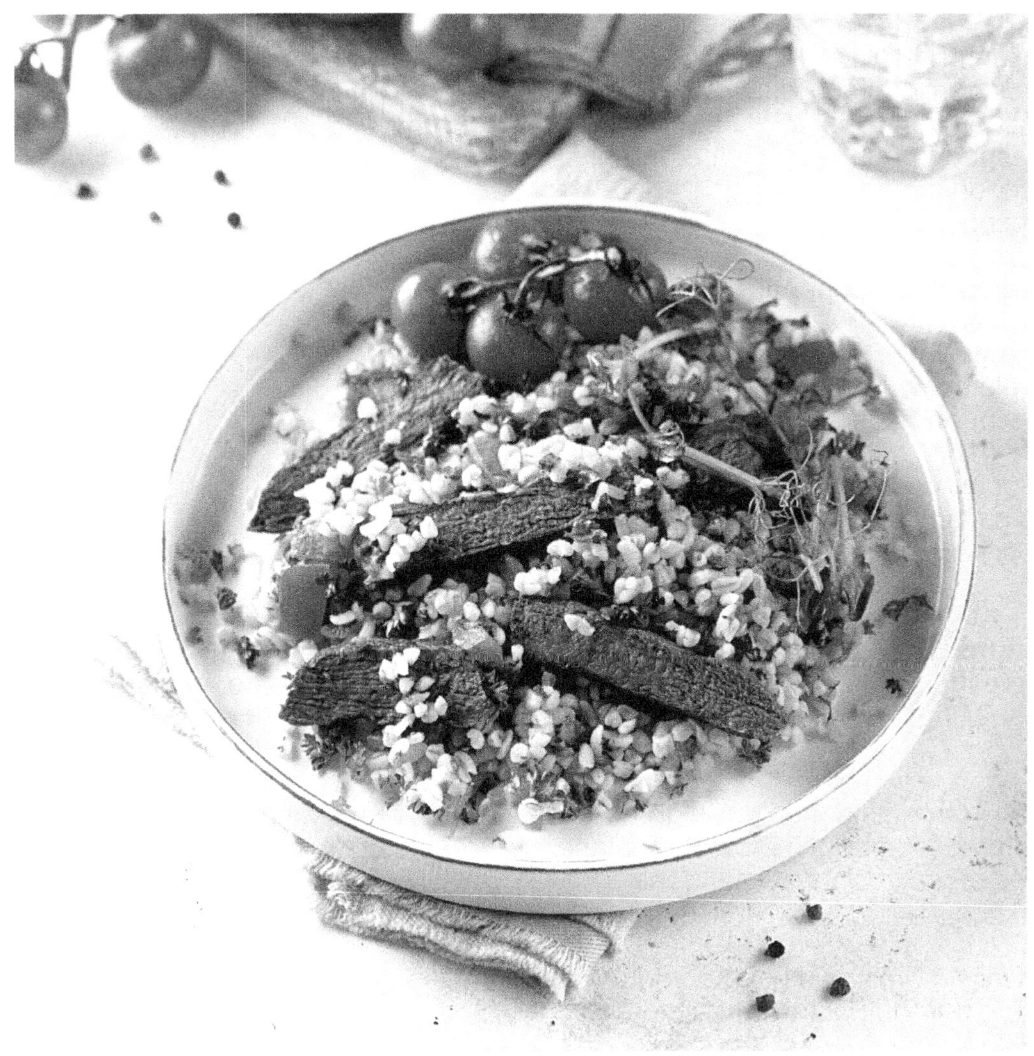

Grilled Chicken Breast with Nutty Yogurt

Yield: 4 Servings
Total Time: 2 Hour 15 Minutes
Prep Time: 5 Minutes
Marinate Time: 2 Hours
Cook Time: 10 Minutes

Ingredients
For the Grilled Chicken:
4 chicken breasts
3 cloves garlic, minced
1 teaspoon cajun spice
1 tablespoon fresh lemon juice, freshly squeezed
1 teaspoon lemon zest
2 tablespoons olive oil
Pinch sea salt
Pinch ground black pepper

For the yogurt:
1 cup plain low-fat Greek yogurt
1 tablespoon fresh lemon juice
1 clove garlic, minced
1 teaspoon fresh basil, roughly chopped
½ cup cucumber, very thinly sliced or shredded
1 cup pistachios, shelled and chopped

Directions
Marinate the chicken in the lemon juice, zest, garlic, cajun spice, and olive oil for roughly 2 hours or overnight in the fridge.

Preheat your grill to medium-high heat. Take out the chicken from the marinade. Lightly grease your grill rack, then place the breasts on top; Cook for about 5 minutes on each side or until done.

Meanwhile, combine all of the yogurt ingredients in a medium bowl. Remember to set aside one-half of the pistachios.

Serve each breast on a large plate. Place a dollop of the nutty yogurt on the side and top the chicken with the remaining pistachios.

Nutritional Information per Serving:
Calories: 460; Total Fat: 21g; Carbs: 11g; Dietary Fiber: 2g; Protein: 55g; Sodium: 254mg

Creamy Mushroom and Leek Risotto

Yield: 4 Servings
Total Time 30 minutes
Prep Time 5 minutes
Cook Time 25 minutes

Ingredients
1 cup Risotto/ Arborio rice
1 leek, thinly sliced
2 cups button mushrooms, sliced
2 tablespoons olive oil
3.5 cups vegetable broth/stock
¼ cup parmesan cheese
¼ cup dry white wine
½ cup parsley, chopped
½ cup coriander, chopped
Pinch salt and pepper

Directions
Heat half olive oil in a large saucepan set over medium heat; sauté mushrooms for about 4 minutes or until browned. Stir in salt and pepper and remove from heat; transfer the mushroom to a dish and set aside.

Return the pan to heat and add the remaining oil; sauté leeks for about 4 minutes or until lightly browned. Stir in rice and cook for about 1 minute. Stir in wine and cook for about 2 minutes or until absorbed.

Ladle in 1 cup of the vegetable broth at a time while stirring until risotto comes back to a simmer. Make sure the risotto does not boil to avoid it getting gummy. Repeat adding in stock and cooking for about 20 minutes or until rice is al dente.

Remove the pan from heat and stir in cheese and two-thirds of the sautéed mushrooms. Stir to coat well and adjust the seasoning.

Serve the risotto topped with the remaining mushrooms, parsley, and coriander.

Nutritional Information per Serving:
Calories: 288; Total Fat: 8.9 g; Net Carbs: 46.4 g; Dietary Fiber: 2.3 g; Sugars: 4.3 g; Protein: 6.3 g; Sodium: 825 mg

Delicious Tofu Curry

Yield: 4 Serving
Total Time: 35 Minutes
Prep Time: 10 Minutes
Cook Time: 25 Minutes

Ingredients
600g (5oz) tofu, diced
400ml (1.7 cups) can light coconut cream
1 teaspoon turmeric
1 small onion
3 cloves garlic
2 tablespoons of Tomato Paste
2 teaspoon curry powder
2 teaspoon of cumin, ground
½ teaspoon cayenne
Pinch of sea salt and pepper

Directions
Add the onion, cayenne, cumin, turmeric, garlic, curry powder, and a tablespoon of water in your food processor, then blend.

Scrape the mixture out of the food processor and into a large saucepan over low heat, add a dash of oil, gently saute for 5 minutes, add the tomato paste and tofu, and increase the heat to high/mid-cook for about 10 minutes stirring.

Add the salt, pepper, and cream; reduce the heat until the curry is simmering. Simmer for 20-25 minutes until the sauce has thickened.

Serve hot with rice of your choice.

Nutritional Information per Serving:
Calories: 214; Total Fat: 14.5 g; Carbs: 8 g; Dietary Fiber: 3 g; Sugars: 4 g; Protein: 12.5 g; Sodium: 55.75 mg

Healthy Green Bean & Zucchini Sauté with Toasted Almonds

Yield: 2 Servings
Total Time: 15 Minutes
Prep Time: 5 Minutes
Cook Time: 10 Minutes

Ingredients
2 tablespoons extra-virgin olive oil
2 cups green beans, sliced
1 cup chopped red onion
2 garlic cloves, minced
Pinch cajun spicy
2 medium zucchini, thinly sliced
A pinch of salt and pepper
2 tablespoons lemon juice
½ cup scallions/spring onions
1 cup sliced toasted almonds

Directions
Add olive oil to a pan set over medium heat.

Stir in red onions for about 5 minutes or until fragrant; add in garlic, green beans, zucchini, cajun spicy, sea salt, and pepper and sauté, stirring, for about 8 minutes or until the veggies are tender.

Remove the pan from heat and stir in lemon juice and spring onions.

Serve topped with sliced toasted almonds.

Nutritional Information per Serving:
Calories: 249; Total Fat: 21.4g; Net Carbs: 17.3g; Dietary Fiber: 7.4g; Sugars: 7g; Protein: 7.5g; Sodium: 185mg

Cheesy Mushroom Omelet

Yield: 3 Servings
Total Time: 10 Minutes
Prep Time: 5 Minutes
Cook Time: 5 Minutes

Ingredients
1 red onion sliced
1 cup sliced button mushrooms
1 zucchini, chopped
1 cup spinach, coarsely chopped
6 eggs
dash of milk
80g (3oz) low-fat cheddar or mozzarella, coarsely grated
25g (0.9oz) of butter
Pinch of salt and pepper

Directions
Preheat oven to 220C/200C fan-forced.

Warm a knob of butter in a non-stick frying pan on medium heat. Add onions and sliced mushrooms and cook, stirring for roughly 3 minutes; add spinach and cook for another 2 minutes until the spinach has slightly wilted. Then transfer to a bowl.

In a large bowl, whisk eggs and a dash of milk. Then add one-third of the low-fat cheddar and whisk again.

Warm the butter in the frying pan again over medium heat; add the cheesy egg mixture.

Cook for a few minutes until the bottom begins to set.

Sprinkle over the mushroom mixture and half the remaining cheddar. Bake for about 3 minutes in the oven or until the omelet is puffed and golden. Sprinkle the remaining cheddar over the omelet. Serve with a sprinkle of fresh basil.

Nutritional Information per Serving:
Calories: 291; Total Fat: 28.4g; Net Carbs: 9g; Dietary Fiber: 1.6g; Sugars: 1.6g; Protein: 23g; Sodium: 185mg

Potato and Leek Soup

Yields: 4 Servings
Total Time: 45 Minutes
Prep Time: 10 Minutes
Cook Time: 35 Minutes

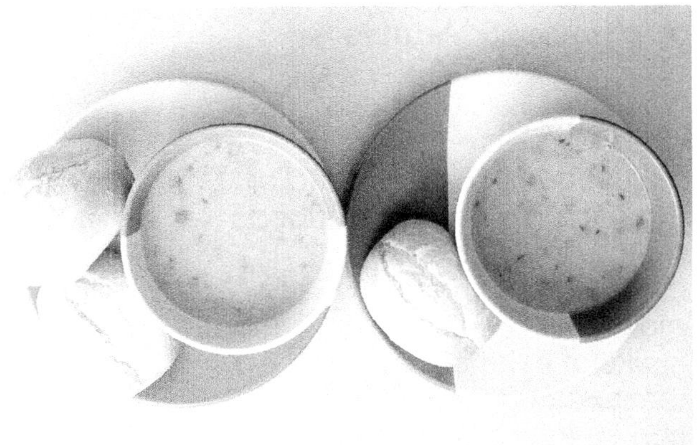

Ingredients

2 tbsp butter
1 large onion, chopped
3 garlic cloves, minced
2 leeks, finely chopped
4 medium potatoes, diced
5 cups chicken or vegetable stock
¾ cup low-fat cream
1 tsp salt and black pepper
1 tsp fresh thyme

Directions

Melt butter in a large pot over medium heat. Add garlic, onion, and leeks and sauté for 5 minutes or until soft and fragrant.

Add stock, then add the diced potatoes. Increase heat and bring to a boil. Then reduce to a simmer, cover with a lid.

Simmer for 25 to 30 minutes or until the potatoes are soft. Remove from heat, and puree with a stick blender. Stir in the cream and season with fresh thyme, salt, and pepper.

Serve, garnished with drizzled with cream and sprinkled with chives.

Nutritional Information per Serving:

Calories: 304; Total Fat: 9g; Net Carbs: 38g; Dietary Fiber: 3.25g; Sugars: 4.7g; Protein: 11g; Sodium: 177mg

Fried Tofu with Greens Beans with Toasted Cashews

Yields: 4 Servings
Total Time: 35 Minutes
Prep Time: 10 Minutes
Cook Time: 25 Minutes

Ingredients
4 tablespoons sesame seed oil
500g (1lb 2oz) firm tofu, cubed
1 red onion, thinly sliced
3 cups of green beans
1 medium red bell pepper, chopped
2 stalks of celery, chopped
2 teaspoons ginger, minced
1 cup spring onions, chopped
2 tablespoons soy sauce
2 tablespoons dry sherry
1 teaspoon maple syrup
1 cup toasted cashews, chopped

Directions
Add half of the oil to a pan set over medium heat. Add tofu and fry until golden. Transfer to a plate.

Add the remaining oil to the pan and sauté the onions until translucent.

Stir in bell pepper, celery and continue to sauté until onions are tender and golden. Stir in ginger, soy sauce, dry sherry, maple syrup, two tablespoons of water and green beans and cook for another few minutes.

Stir in the tofu and season; simmer until warmed through, then serve. Top with chopped toasted cashews.

Nutritional Information per Serving:
Calories: 294; Total Fat: 16g; Net Carbs: 24g; Dietary Fiber: 6g; Sugars: 10.3g; Protein: 17.3g; Sodium: 477mg

Superfood Nutty Collard Wraps

Yield: 4 Servings
Total Time: 15 Minutes
Prep Time: 15 Minutes
Cook Time: N/A

Ingredients
4 collard leaves (Brassica oleracea)
1 cup toasted almonds, chopped
1 ripe avocado, sliced
1 cup alfalfa sprouts
1 red bell pepper, sliced
1 yellow pepper, sliced
1 lemon
2 tablespoon extra-virgin olive oil
1 teaspoon cumin
1 teaspoon grated ginger
1 tablespoon light soy sauce
1 lime

Directions
Remove the stems from the collard leaves and rinse them under running cold water to remove any grit and dirt.

Soak the collard leaves in lemon juice and warm water for about 8 minutes, then dry using paper towels.

Add the toasted nuts, cumin, light soy sauce, ginger, and olive oil to your food processor. Pulse until the mixture forms a soft ball-like shape.

Layout the collard leaves and divide the nutty almond mix among the leaves. Top with sliced red and yellow pepper, avocado, alfalfa sprouts, and drizzle lemon juice on top and sprinkle with salt and pepper. Fold in the top and bottom parts, then roll up the sides.

Slice the wrap in two, if desired, and serve immediately.

Nutritional Information per Serving:
Calories: 143; Total Fat: 9g; Net Carbs: 11.2g; Dietary Fiber: 3g; Sugars: 4.5g; Protein: 3g; Sodium: 99.34mg

Vegan Ratatouille

Yield: 4 Servings
Total Time: 1 Hour 20 Minutes
Prep Time: 20 Minutes
Cook Time: 1 Hour

Ingredients
1 tablespoon extra-virgin olive oil
1 can (400g/14oz) crushed tomatoes
½ teaspoon chili powder
1 teaspoon Italian seasoning
1 tablespoon chopped fresh basil
1 teaspoon minced garlic
¼ teaspoon salt and pepper
2 red onions, chopped
4 large fresh tomatoes, sliced
1 large eggplant, sliced
2 large zucchinis, sliced
1 yellow bell pepper, sliced

Directions
Preheat your oven to 350°F/177°C and lightly grease a baking dish.

Mix together crushed tomatoes, chili powder, Italian seasoning, basil, garlic, and salt in a bowl and pour the mixture into the prepared baking dish.

Layer vegetable slices on top of the tomato mixture in rows until you have used all the veggies. Spray the veggies with oil and season with salt and pepper; bake in the oven for about 1 hour or until the tomato sauce is bubbly and veggies tender. Serve hot garnished with fresh chopped basil.

Nutritional Information per Serving:
Calories: 318; Total Fat: 1g; Net Carbs: 52g; Dietary Fiber: 10.7g; Sugars: 27g; Protein: 16g; Sodium: 350mg

Chicken Stir Fry with Avocado & Red Onions

Yield: 4 Servings
Total Time: 20 Minutes
Prep Time: 10 Minutes
Cook Time: 10 Minutes

Ingredients:
450g (1lb) skinless chicken breasts, thinly sliced strips
2 tablespoons balsamic vinegar
Pinch of sea salt and pepper
4 tablespoons sesame seed oil
2 tablespoons of maple syrup
1 tablespoon wholegrain mustard
1 large red onion, thinly chopped
1 red bell pepper, thinly sliced
1 green bell pepper, thinly sliced
1 tablespoon toasted sesame seeds
1 teaspoon crushed red pepper flakes
4 cups cabbage
1 avocado, diced

Directions:
Place chicken in a bowl; stir in balsamic vinegar, maple syrup, red pepper flakes, mustard, sesame seed oil, salt, and pepper. Toss to coat well.

Heat a tablespoon of sesame oil in a pan set over medium-high heat; add chicken and cook for about 5 minutes or until chicken is browned, then rcmove from heat.

Heat the remaining oil to the pan and sauté onions for about 2 minutes or until caramelized; stir in red and green peppers and cook for 3 minutes more.

Stir in cabbage and cook for 2 minutes; return chicken to the pan and stir in sesame seeds . Serve hot topped with diced avocado!

Nutritional Info Per Serving:
Calories: 437; Fat: 24g; Carbs: 16.25g; Dietary Fiber: 3.5g; Sugars: 7.8 g; Protein: 38g; Sodium: 166mg

Turmeric Chickpea & Artichoke Sauté Wraps

Yield: 4 Servings
Total Time: 15 Minutes
Prep Time: 5 Minutes
Cook Time: 10 Minutes

Ingredients
3 tablespoons extra virgin olive oil
1 ½ cups artichoke hearts
2 cups cooked chickpeas
1 small brown onion
1 tablespoon minced garlic
½ cup fresh coriander, chopped
2 teaspoons turmeric
½ teaspoon paprika
1 teaspoon ginger, minced
Pinch sea salt and black pepper
4 multi-grain wraps

Directions
Heat a pan over medium to high heat; add spices, garlic, onion, ginger, and olive oil.

Then toss in artichoke hearts, chickpeas, and season with salt and pepper; Stir for about 6 minutes or until chickpeas are browned. Serve drizzled with fresh lemon juice, and sprinkle fresh coriander in multi-grain wraps.

Nutrition Information per Serving:
Calories: 654; Total Fat: 19.2g; Net Carbs: 108g; Dietary Fiber: 25.1g; Sugars: 17g Protein: 27g; Sodium: 765mg

Grilled Lemon Chicken & Chicory-Orange Salad with Ginger Dressing

Yield: 4 Servings
Total Time: 25 Minutes
Prep Time: 10 Minutes
Cook Time: 15 Minutes

Ingredients
For the dressing
¼ cup olive oil
1 teaspoon honey
2 tablespoons fresh lemon juice
1 tablespoon orange juice
½ teaspoon finely grated orange zest
1 teaspoon American mustard
1 garlic clove, crushed
1 teaspoon freshly grated ginger

For the salad
500g (1lb 1.7oz) skinless, boneless chicken breasts
4 tablespoons fresh lemon juice
A pinch of salt and pepper
1 cup rocket, chopped
3 cups lettuce, chopped
1 large head of chicory, chopped
1 orange, peeled, segmented, and deseeded

Directions
Dressing: In a jar, combine all dressing ingredients and shake to mix well. Chill in the refrigerator for at least 1 hour before using.

Then combine all salad ingredients in a large bowl and chill.

Meanwhile, whisk together lemon juice, salt, and pepper until well combined; add in chicken breasts and toss to coat well.

Place on a preheated charcoal grill and cook for about 8 minutes per side or until cooked through and golden brown.

Serve the salad drizzled with the dressing and toss to coat well. Top each serving with grilled chicken.

Nutritional Info Per Serving:
Calories: 381; Fat: 18g; Carbs: 12.6 g; Dietary Fiber: 4.75g; Sugars: 6g; Protein: 39g; Sodium: 105mg

BBQ Chicken with Healthy Almond & Pistachio Pesto

Yield: 4 Servings
Total Time: 15 Minutes
Prep Time: 10 Minutes
Cook Time: 5 Minutes

Ingredients
4 (150g/ 5.3oz) chicken breasts
1 tablespoon extra-virgin olive oil
1 red bell pepper, chopped
1 cup baby Spinach
1 cup rocket

Almond & Pistachio pesto
½ cup extra-virgin olive oil
½ cup toasted pistachios
¼ cup toasted almonds
½ fresh lime, juiced
pinch of red chili flakes
2 garlic cloves
½ cup basil leaves
½ cup mint leaves
½ cup baby rocket

Directions
In a food processor, process fresh lime juice, toasted pistachios, almonds, garlic, chili, basil, rocket, and mint until smooth, add oil, salt, and pepper, and continue pulsing until very smooth. Set aside.

Preheat the BBQ grill on medium heat, and then brush the chicken with oil and season with salt and pepper.

Grill for about 8 minutes per side or until the chicken is cooked. Transfer to a plate.

Slice the chicken and divide among the serving plates; top each serving with spinach and red bell pepper and season with salt and pepper.

Serve with the creamy almond and pistachio pesto.

Nutritional Information per Serving:
Calories: 461; Total Fat: 24.5g; Net Carbs: 8.7g; Dietary Fiber: 3.75g; Sugars: 4g; Protein: 51g; Sodium: 179mg

Best Roast Potatoes

Yield: 4 Servings
Total Time: 25 Minutes
Prep Time: 5 Minutes
Steam Time: 5 to 8 Minutes
Roast Time: 30 Minutes

Ingredients

1kg(2lb 3.3oz) potatoes, peeled and quartered
Canola oil, spray
1 tablespoon fresh rosemary, chopped
1 teaspoon fresh thyme.
1 tsp salt and pepper

Directions

Steam the washed cut potatoes until just undercooked. Then transfer to a bowl and roughly shake the potatoes till fluffy but not falling apart.

Arrange the fluffy potatoes on a baking tray. Spray with canola oil and season with salt, pepper, thyme, and rosemary.

Bake in preheated oven 482°F/ 250°C for 25 to 30 minutes or until golden and crispy.

Nutritional Information per Serving:

Calories: 275; Total Fat: 2g; Carbs: 65g; Dietary Fiber: 5g; Sugars: 2.5g; Protein: 7.5g; Sodium: 136mg

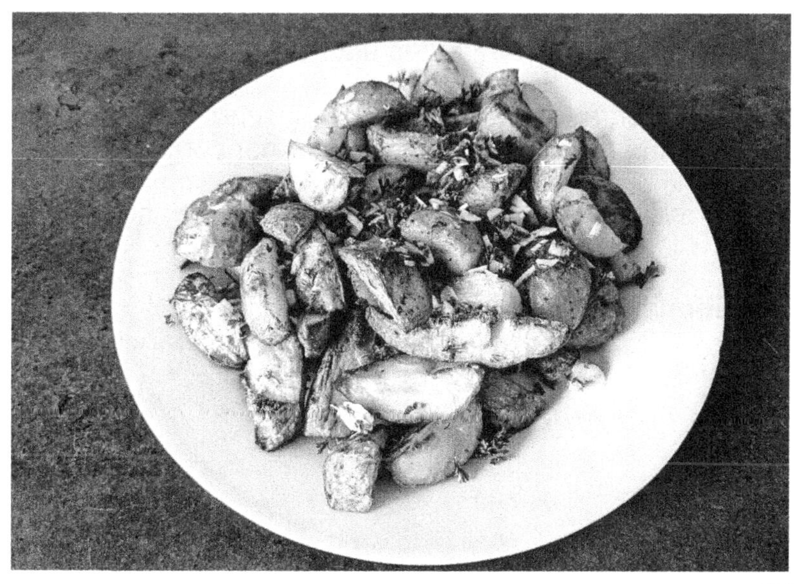

Spicy Coconut Lentil Soup with Rice

Yield: 4 Servings
Total Time: 45 Minutes
Prep Time: 15 Minutes
Cook Time: 30 Minutes

Ingredients
4 cups vegetable broth
1 large onion, diced
1 ½ cups red lentils, soaked
1 tablespoon garlic, minced
1 teaspoon ginger, minced
1 teaspoon lemongrass paste
2 tablespoons tomato paste
1 cup light coconut milk
1 tablespoon curry powder
Pinch of salt and pepper
1 cup hot cooked rice of your choice
fresh cilantro/coriander

Directions
Heat a dash of oil in a large pot over medium heat. Add the onion, ginger, and garlic and cook until soft and fragrant.

Add the curry powder, tomato paste, lemongrass paste, and fry, constantly stirring, for 30 seconds to release the aroma.

Add the lentils and vegetable broth. Raise the heat to bring it to a boil then cover and reduce the heat to a simmer.

Simmer for about 30 minutes until the lentils are tender.

Once tender, add the cooked rice, coconut milk, salt, and pepper. Raise the heat to medium and allow to cook for another couple of minutes until hot.

Serve the soup hot, garnished with fresh coriander/cilantro.

Nutritional Information per Serving:
Calories: 332; Total Fat: 4g; Carbs: 58g; Dietary Fiber: 9.2g; Sugars: 4.5g; Protein: 17.5g; Sodium: 749mg

No Yeast Pizza Dough

Yield: 4 Servings
Total Time: 25 Minutes
Prep Time: 10 Minutes
Cook Time: 15 Minutes

Makes 2 Pizzas

Ingredients
2 ½ cups plain flour
2 tsp baking powder
¼ cup parmesan cheese
2 tablespoons vegetable oil
⅔ cup warm water

Directions
Mix all the dry ingredients in a large bowl. Make a well, then add warm water and oil. Mix well; then knead for 3 to 4 minutes.

Cover in plastic wrap and set aside somewhere warm, and prepare your pizza topping.

Sprinkle your work surface with extra flour, then roll out the pizza dough.

Add whatever topping you choose. Bake for roughly 12 minutes until the edges are crispy and golden.

Nutritional Information per Serving:
Calories: 360; Total Fat: 8.5g; Carbs: 59g; Dietary Fiber: 2g; Sugars: 1.5g; Protein: 9.5g; Sodium: 133mg

Garlic Lemon Spaghetti

Yield: 2 Serving
Total Time: 25 Minutes
Prep Time: 25 Minutes
Cook Time: N/A

Ingredients
340g (12 oz) dried spaghetti
4 tablespoons olive oil
1 tablespoon butter
1 tablespoon minced garlic
½ teaspoon red pepper flakes or more
1 large lemon juice and zest
½ cup chopped fresh parsley
½ cup fresh basil leaves
Pinch salt and black pepper
50g (2 oz) parmesan cheese freshly grated

Directions
Cook spaghetti as per packet instructions. Meanwhile, heat olive oil in a large frying pan over medium heat. Add minced garlic and red pepper flakes; cook and stir until fragrant. Remove from heat.

Once you've drained the spaghetti, warm the large frying pan with the garlic mixture over medium heat. Add drained, cooked spaghetti and ¼ cup of reserved pasta water; toss to coat. Cook and stir until hot. Add more spaghetti water if it seems too dry.

Remove the spaghetti from heat. Stir in butter, basil, parsley, lemon juice, and zest—season with salt and pepper. Transfer to serving bowls; top with grated parmesan cheese and serve.

Nutrition Information per Serving
Calories: 630; Total Fat: 34g; Carbs: 60g; Dietary Fiber: 5g; Sugars: 3.5g; Protein: 13g; Sodium: 317mg

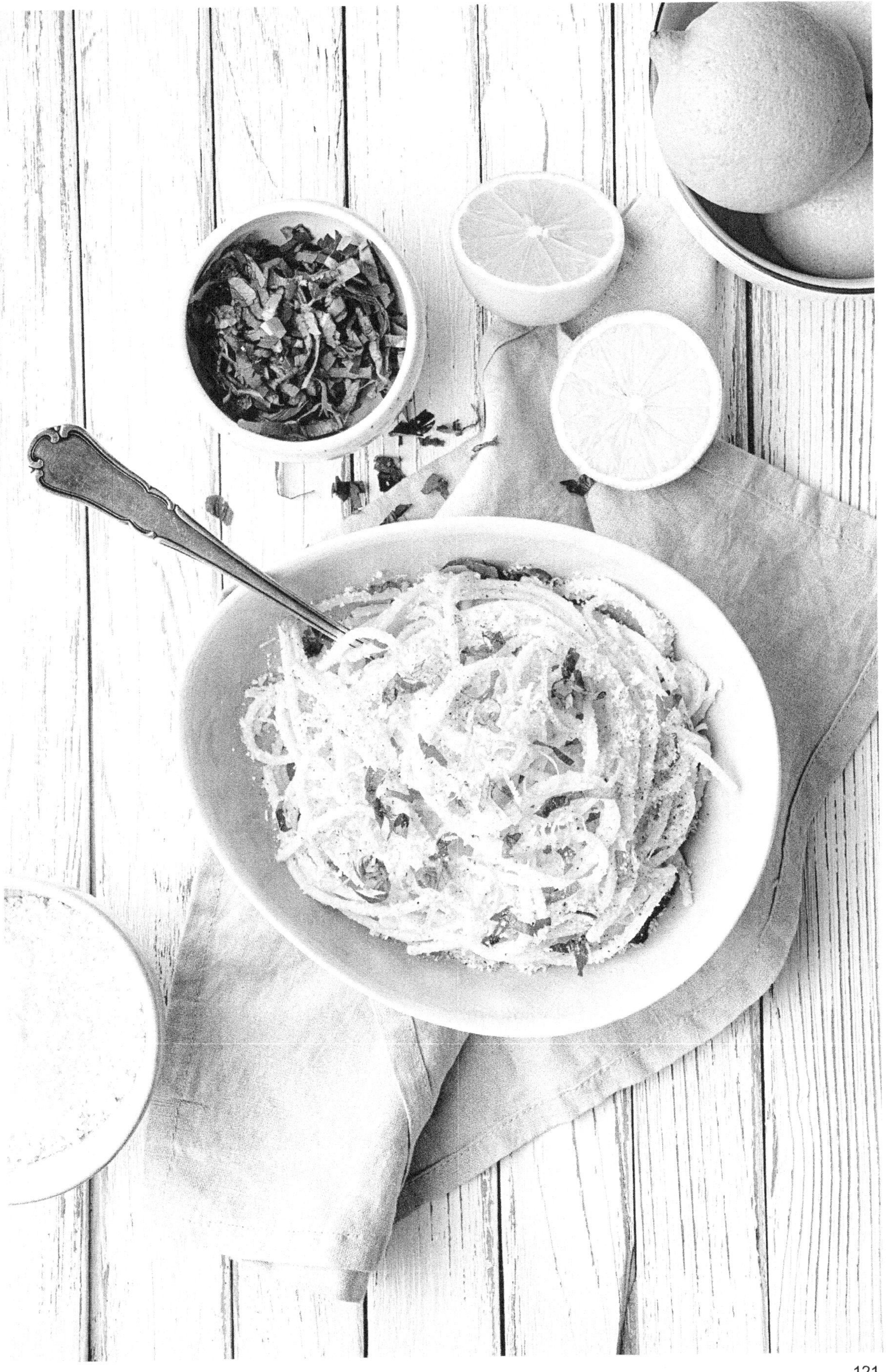

Butternut Squash Pasta Sauce

Yield: 5 Servings
Total Time: 85 Minutes
Prep Time: 25 Minutes
Cook Time: 60 Minutes

Ingredients
1 butternut squash
450g (1lb) pasta
2 tablespoons extra-virgin olive oil
1 onion, chopped
3 garlic cloves
½ cup grated Parmesan cheese
⅓ cup low-fat Greek yogurt
2 tablespoon chopped parsley for garnish
2 tablespoons, chopped basil
Pinch salt and pepper
1 to 2 cups veggie broth to thin the sauce

Directions
Preheat the oven at 350°F/180°C. Peel and chop the butternut squash into large cubes.

Pour 1/2 cup of veggie broth into a baking dish and place the cubed butternut squash on top; cover with foil. Bake for roughly 35 minutes or until a fork easily pierces the squash. Allow cooling for 10 minutes.

Once cooled, blend in a blender.

In a pan, saute the onions and garlic with olive oil for about 3 minutes. Then add the onions and garlic to the blender with 1/2 cup of veggie broth, parmesan cheese, and season with salt and pepper.

If the sauce is too thick, thin it a little more with more veggie broth.

Pour the sauce into a saucepan and set over a low heat. Stir in the Greek yogurt and warm it through.

In the meantime, cook pasta in boiling salted water. Once the pasta is cooked; drain and pour into a large bowl. Then pour the butternut sauce over the pasta and stir.

Serve hot. Garnish with chopped basil and parsley.

Nutritional Information per Serving:
Calories: 568; Total Fat: 8.5g; Carbs: 106g; Dietary Fiber: 8g; Sugars: 11g; Protein: 20g; Sodium: 103mg

Snacks

"Cooking is love made visible."

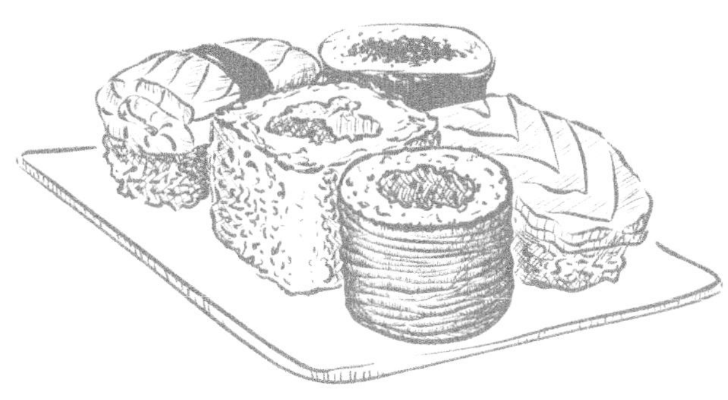

Nutty Turmeric & Coconut Balls

Yield: 12 Servings
Total Time: 10 Minutes
Prep Time: 10 Minutes
Cook Time: N/A

Ingredients
½ cup raw cashews
½ cup walnuts
1 ½ cup shredded coconut
1 tablespoon pumpkin seeds
2 tablespoon maple syrup
3 teaspoons ground turmeric
1 teaspoon cinnamon
1 teaspoon ground ginger
1 teaspoon black pepper
½ teaspoon salt

Directions
In a blender, blend coconut until almost oily. This can take quite a long time, but it is important to wait until the coconut starts to stick to the sides; add the rest of the ingredients and process until cashews and walnuts are finely chopped. Press the mixture into bite-sized balls and arrange them on a baking tray. Refrigerate until firm before serving.

Nutritional Information per Serving:
Calories: 104; Total Fat: 7g; Net Carbs: 8.3g; Dietary Fiber: 1.3g: Sugars: 4.5g; Protein: 2.2g; Sodium: 32.6mg

Roasted Chili-Vinegar Peanuts

Yield: 4 Servings
Total Time: 20 Minutes
Prep Time: 5 Minutes
Cook Time: 15 Minutes

Ingredients
1 tablespoon coconut oil
2 cups raw peanuts, unsalted
2 teaspoon sea salt
½ teaspoon black pepper
2 tablespoon apple cider vinegar
1 teaspoon chili powder
1 ½ teaspoons fresh lime zest

Directions

Preheat oven to 350°F/177°C

In a large bowl, toss together coconut oil, peanuts, black pepper, and salt until well coated.

Transfer to a rimmed baking sheet and roast in the oven for about 15 minutes or until fragrant.

Transfer the roasted peanuts to a bowl and add vinegar, chili powder, and lime zest.

Toss to coat well and serve.

Nutritional Information per Serving:
Calories: 427; Total Fat: 37.5g; Net Carbs: 8g; Dietary Fiber: 6.5g; Sugars: 3g; Protein: 18.9g; Sodium: 156mg

Tangy and Salted Carrot and Parsnip French Fries

Yield: 4 Servings
Total Time: 35 Minutes
Prep Time: 15 Minutes
Cook Time: 20 Minutes

Ingredients
6 large carrots
4 large parsnips
2 tablespoons extra virgin olive oil
½ teaspoon sea salt
½ teaspoon of pepper
2 tablespoons fresh lemon juice
1 tablespoon freshly chopped basil

Directions
Chop the carrots and parsnips into 3-inch sections and then cut each section into thin sticks.

Toss together the carrots and parsnip sticks with extra virgin olive oil, lemon juice in a large bowl. Then spread into a baking sheet lined with parchment paper, sprinkle with salt and pepper.

Bake the sticks at 425°F/218°C for about 20 minutes or until browned. Top with freshly chopped basil leaves and serve.

Nutritional Information per Serving:
Calories: 212; Total Fat: 7.25g;Net Carbs: 36.2g; Dietary Fiber: 10g Sugars: 5g; Protein: 3.8g; Sodium: 219mg

Zucchini Muffins

Yield: 6 muffins
Total Time: 35 Minutes
Prep Time: 10 Minutes
Cook Time: 25 Minutes

Ingredients
1 brown onion
2 zucchini, grated
2 cups (300g) self-raising flour
1 cup (150g) light cheddar cheese, grated
1 small chili pepper (deseeded) finely chopped
2 Eggs
¾ cup (185ml) semi skimmed milk
60g butter, melted
Pinch salt and pepper

Directions
Preheat oven to 355°F/ 180°C. Line a muffin pan with paper cases.

Pan fry onions over medium heat for about 5 minutes or until the onions are soft. Set aside to cool.

Combine the zucchini, flour, cheddar, chili, salt, and pepper in a large bowl. Add the onions and stir to combine.

In another bowl, whisk the eggs, milk, and butter; pour the egg mixture into the zucchini bowl and stir until combined.

Spoon evenly into the lined muffin pan. Bake for 25 mins or until a skewer inserted in the center comes out clean.

Nutritional Information per Serving:
Calories: 355; Total Fat: 12g; Carbs: 41g; Dietary Fiber: 2.5g; Sugars: 6g; Protein: 16.6g; Sodium: 108mg

Easy Cherry, Oaty Balls

Yield: 15 balls
Total Time: 70 Minutes
Prep Time: 10 Minutes
Chill Time: 60 Minutes

Ingredients
10 fresh dates, seeded, coarsely chopped
1 cup (90g) rolled oats
¼ cup (40g) dried cherries
¼ cup (50g) pumpkin seeds, toasted
2 tbsp almond butter

Directions
Blend the dates in a blender until smooth, then transfer to a medium bowl.

Add the oats, cherries, sunflower seeds, and almond butter and stir until well combined.

Using wet hands, roll the date mixture into small balls. Place onto a baking sheet on a tray. Chill in the refrigerator for at least an hour, then store in an airtight container.

Nutritional Information per Serving:
Calories: 65; Total Fat: 2.9g; Carbs: 9g; Dietary Fiber: 1g; Sugars: 5.6g; Protein: 1.8g; Sodium: 24mg

Healthy Party Sushi

Yield: 48 slices
Total Time: 45 Minutes
Prep Time: 35 Minutes
Cook Time: 15 Minutes
Serve size is 4 slices each

Ingredients
2 ½ cups (500g) sushi rice, rinsed, drained
½ cup (125ml) rice wine vinegar
3 teaspoons caster sugar
½ teaspoon, salt
6 nori sheets
1 cucumber, cut into strips
1 red bell pepper, cut into strips
1 avocado, cut into batons
Pickled Jalapenos, finely chopped
Salt-reduced soy sauce, to serve

Directions
Cook the sushi rice as per the pack instructions.

Combine the vinegar, jalapenos, sugar, and salt in a small bowl. Transfer the rice to a large bowl, then slowly fold the vinegar mixture into the bowl. Make sure to break up any rice clumps. Allow the rice to cool.

Place a bamboo sushi mat on a clean work surface with the slats running horizontally. Place 1 nori sheet, shiny side down, on the mat. Spread a portion of rice over the nori sheet, leaving a 3cm-wide border along the edge furthest from you.

Place the cucumber strips, red bell pepper, and avocado along the center of the rice. Holding the filling in place, roll the mat over to enclose rice and filling. Repeat with remaining nori, rice, and fillings. Cut each roll into approximately 8 slices. Serve with soy sauce for dipping.

Nutritional Information per Serving:
Calories: 109; Total Fat: 2.4g; Carbs: 20g; Dietary Fiber: 1.5g; Sugars: 2.2g; Protein: 1.5g; Sodium: 450mg

Made in the USA
Middletown, DE
20 April 2022

64556602R00073